191333

# Alzheimer's

## It will never be all right!

### by Patti Grose

Library of Congress Control Number: 2005902871

ISBN 0-9767702-0-2

Cover, text design, sketches and photographs by Patti Grose

Printed in the United States of America

10  9  8  7  6  5  4  3  2  1

Signature Book Printing, Inc.
Gaithersburg, MD 20879

Edited by Barbara Marinelli

Published by Lovespun Treasures, LLC
Highland, MD 20777
www.lovespuntreasures.com

806-H
c.1

Deciding to "write a book" is a grand idea. Writing a book is another thing entirely. I could not have made this humble attempt if it were not for having so much support. I would like to acknowledge my loving family, Ray (my faithful partner), Matthew, JR, Karen, Kelsey, Kayla, Chris, and Scott and my two sisters, Jean and Joy, for being a part of *my* story.

I am thankful for very dear friends: Thank you to Mary and Joe Rekus for your friendship, encouragement and always being there and to Cathy Walsh for your friendship, encouragement and introducing me to Barbara.

I am also thankful for new friends: Thank you to Barbara Marinelli for your insightful editing skills, asking the right questions and for your time that allowed us to get to know one another and to Trudy Mathews for your willingness to be the "stranger to read my writing" and for encouraging me to share my story.

The list of others to whom I offer my gratitude include: The professionals for your dedication, skill and kindness in caring for Charlotte—

Respite Care: Yolanda, Linda and Diane

Western Howard Senior Plus: Judy, Audrey, Lynn and Rose

Winter Growth Adult Day Care Center: Cyndi, Kathy, Karen, Monique, Glory, Donna, Evelyne, Fatou, Jennie, Jim, Joelle, Laura, Shari, Sue, Shirley, Barbara, Connie, Charlotte and Emma

Howard County Department on Aging: Darlene, Marsha, Betty, Xiomara and Ernestine

Howard County Health Department: Jeanne and Carolyn

Autumn Hill Assisted-Living Residence: Victoria, Bunny, Ann, Meg, Mary, Tamara and Louisa

Charlotte's doctors: Macharan, Fish, Rosenberg and Beth Gallagher, RN, MSN, CRNP for your service dedicated to Charlotte's well-being.

Mary Ann Wilkerson, EdD, APRN, PMH—Humanim, for your time and insightful comments. I needed them.

Website: Damar Group, Ltd. for e-business solutions

*This book is dedicated to*

*...our Charlotte*

*and to others like*

*...Julia and Jack*
*...Chris and Stan*
*...Kate and Ray*

*living their own stories of Alzheimer's.*

# Table of Contents

# *Preface*

This story is taken from a caregiver's journal in which a family member develops Alzheimer's. It is a story, sometimes solemn, sometimes funny—a heartfelt assessment to share with others who are going through this crisis in their lives. It also tells of the relationship between a mother-in-law and daughter-in-law and how that relationship has been affected by Charlotte having Alzheimer's disease.

Hopefully, it will bring a message of understanding, hope and worthy advice to the reader. Charlotte would love to know that she is the topic of a book. The heroine of our story is now in the latter stages of Alzheimer's and still an important part of our family.

*Living with Alzheimer's...*
    *an ordinary family's story*

# ♥ *Chapter One...*

## *Background*
### *"Who we are...from my perspective"*

I met Charlotte when I was thirteen years old. Her son, Ray, was my first and only true love. He introduced us. He brought me to meet Charlotte one evening after our Teen Center Dance. I remember her being so young.

Immediately after our introduction, Charlotte proudly stated that she was 36 years old and that when she was younger, she had the exact body measurements of some famous movie star of her generation. (I believe it was the 1959 Miss America, Mary Ann Mobley, who Charlotte, with such delight, said that she replicated.) She even

1

told me that her husband was fourteen years older than she and that he worked in the evenings. Her choice of topics seemed very strange to me. My mother would have been asking if we were hungry and stating all of the choices she could prepare for us—finding out just what we liked. My mom was thirty-five when she gave birth to me, her fourth daughter and last child. She was not into glamour; I had unconsciously assumed that most mothers were like mine, and Charlotte did not seem to be like my Mom.

Another thing I found different that first evening—plastic slipcovers on her furniture! Ray's mom (as I have referred to her most of our lives) was from a different mold than what I knew as "mother." I tell you this right up front, so you will know that, from my perspective, Ray's mom was not like other moms I knew; from the very beginning it was not "love at first sight."

Having been raised with a strong emphasis on respecting adults or at least acting with respect toward them, this was the relationship I had with Ray's mom from the start. I acted respectfully toward her. Ray's mom was more interested in what I was wearing and how I looked than who I was. She said very complimentary things about my physical appearance and not much about my personality, as I remember.

In contrast, one of my mother's favorite statements, "beauty is as beauty

2

does," made it clear to me that who you were was much more important than what you looked like.

As I got to know Ray's family better, I judged that Charlotte was very much like her stoic, self-focused German mother. If I even mentioned to Charlotte that she reminded me of her mother, she did not like it. I guess she wanted to be told that she was more like her father who was warm, personable and dearly loved by all of the family.

Ray's dad, Art, was friendly and so much fun. It was love at first sight for me with Ray's dad. He played a guitar, sang, and told jokes. I really liked him and enjoyed his cutting up. He wanted to know who I was and what I liked to do and what I saw in his son!

By the time that Ray and I had become teenage sweethearts, my dad and Ray's dad had become best friends. They were both veterans of WWII and had much in common. It was great that the love and friendship that Ray and I had found was also discovered in the relationship between our fathers.

Our dads' close friendship fostered our parents getting together for cards and attending bull roasts and crab feasts. Ray's mom and dad came to my parents' home for all of the holiday celebrations as my mom had a very welcoming way and her mantra, "the more, the merrier," was lived out. My mother never spoke ill of anyone, so I did

3

not say anything to her about my negative reaction to Charlotte.

Ray's dad died in 1968. This was two weeks before our first child, JR, turned one. It happened suddenly on Mother's Day. Ray's mom and dad and Ray and I were laughing and enjoying JR. Right in front of our very eyes, Dad had a cerebral hemorrhage. He died the next day. We were all in the state of shock.

My dad took Art's death very hard; they had seen each other almost daily. Ray's dad was dearly loved for his warm, friendly, down-home West Virginia personality. He was taken so quickly and without any real warning that all of us just seemed to go through the daily motions of life in disbelief.

Charlotte was 44 years old. Her strong, independent nature seemed to allow her to weather this loss.

Knowing that I need to keep on track is a struggle for me; I get side-tracked and give you unnecessary tidbits. Saying that, I realize that you may need a little background on who I am—who I think I am anyway—for you to put the pieces together.

So here goes: I believe I must start with who I am as I am telling you our story.

I am an extravert and have a catalyst-type nature. I am very family oriented, the youngest of four sisters (second oldest died of lung cancer in 2001); my mother and father are deceased. My husband, Ray, is my best friend and confidant. Ray is selfless and the quiet, unassuming worker behind the scenes. He is an introvert with a quick wit and a great, dry sense of humor. We have two sons, JR and Matthew. JR's lovely wife, Karen, came into our family with her two fine sons, Chris and Scott. A year and a half later, our first granddaughter, Kelsey, was born and Kayla came eighteen months later. We are a blessed family.

I taught Kindergarten until my dad came to live with us in 1990 and needed full-time care. Being at home with Daddy, I had time to become an avid gardener and consummate volunteer. Daddy was with us until his death in 1993.

I am a doer. I am a questioner. I seek out other people's experiences to draw information for my own decision-making and to verify that what I feel in my gut is the right way to go. Give me a problem or concern and I gladly tackle the challenge. I take on a stranger's dilemma as quickly and eagerly as one of a dear friend or family member. It makes me feel so worthwhile to find answers and to offer suggestions and solutions.

Sometimes, I can take on too much and become grouchy and impolite to those closest to me, the ones I love the most. I can become consumed by the latest crisis, have a very hard time setting boundaries, become too involved and have difficulty letting go. After a difficult challenge or time of crisis passes, I can crash and not be able to do anything for days.

At times, spontaneity gets me into hot water. Now and then, I can accurately be accused of acting before thinking an action through. My expectations of others are high and even higher for myself, and I struggle with being judgmental of those around me. I am driven to try to achieve perfection, an unwanted vice.

The highest compliment that someone can give me is that I accomplished something to make it easier or better for him or her, thus the reason for sharing with you about our journey with Alzheimer's.

I am ever striving to be closer to God and do my part to be of service to others in my own little part of the world.

# ♥ Chapter Two...

## Charlotte

*"Charlotte is the reason for telling this story."*

Charlotte is the reason for telling this story.

Charlotte was married twice and had several men friends after being widowed two times. She had worked a good part of her married life, primarily as a billing clerk and then as a receptionist at a local hospital. She applied for a secretarial job in the cardiac intensive care unit and unofficially got the job until it was discovered that she had only finished the ninth grade. To qualify for the job, she needed to be a high school graduate. At age 54, she went to classes and received her GED. Everyone was impressed with her drive and commitment. She landed this high-pressured, demanding job and held it until her retirement at age 62.

Charlotte was meticulous, very conscientious about her grooming, the way she kept house and the way she managed her finances. She never had a debt she did not or could not pay.

Five months after Ray's dad died, Charlotte married a long-time family friend. He had lost his wife the month before Ray's dad died. Our relationship with Charlotte and her second husband was barely cordial to say the least. It was not until our second son was born three years later that we began to see Ray's mom on a more regular basis. When Matthew was ten hours old, all of his vital signs plummeted, and the doctor told us that he might not live through the night. Ray called his mom to let her know. She came to the hospital and showed great concern for her new grandson. It seemed that this crisis brought us closer. When we learned that our precious son was going to live, we were so grateful and happy. It was now so much easier to let go of past discord and celebrate our little miracle, Matthew. We kept in much better contact thereafter.

This second marriage lasted for several years and ended with a separation but no divorce. This husband died in the 1980s, leaving Charlotte once again officially widowed.

Charlotte sold her home and moved into a lovely apartment. She was still working at the hospital fulltime and leading a very active social life.

Charlotte dated several men during this period. My favorite was our next-door neighbor, Mr. Joe. Playing the matchmaker, I fixed them up. Our entire family loved Mr. Joe. His wife had died after a long illness three years before he and Charlotte started dating. Mr. Joe was so good to her and for her. He seemed to bring out the best in Charlotte. They had great times dancing and going to the beach, two things she truly loved. Their relationship was fun and loving and lasted until Mr. Joe died several years later.

Charlotte retired from her hospital job and got a part-time job at a fast food restaurant as a welcoming hostess. She loved it as she could dress up and meet people.

One important characteristic of Charlotte that I have not mentioned yet is her love of jewelry. When our Matthew was a little boy, he called his grandmother "Mrs. T," because she reminded him of the TV character, Mr. T, who wore oodles of gold chains and other jewelry. It truly was a great description. Charlotte had five holes pierced in each ear so she could wear more earrings. She had at least one ring on each finger, a couple on her toes, bracelets galore and wore as many necklaces as she could at one time. Ray's dad would call Charlotte "the crow," saying that she went after anything that sparkled! Most people could not help but comment on her jewelry and she loved all of the attention. Charlotte often told us how much everyone admired her jewelry, and fussed over her appearance.

Many times Charlotte told me, "One day, all my jewelry will be yours!" I would jokingly reply that I would have to grow more arms than an octopus to accommodate all of her jewelry! She would giggle, and I would smile sheepishly, as I thought about how much jewelry she actually had.

In 1995, Charlotte was hospitalized several times in a short period with symptoms of shortness of breath, dizziness and chest pains; each time Charlotte was sent home. Finally, it was decided that she was having anxiety attacks. She reluctantly did admit to us that she was having a difficult time financially. This must have been very hard for this self-sufficient woman, who had been on her own for so long, to reveal—even to her son and me. I asked Ray if it was time to extend an invitation to her to come and live with us.

I readily admit to being my mother's child in that her example of taking care of family members was what I had known from childhood. I was thinking of how good Ray was to my dad when he was unable to live on his own anymore and came to live with us. Ray is an only child, so there was no one else to consult or with whom to share Charlotte's fate. It just seemed that now was the time for us to care for his mom and for us to make her this offer. Ray agreed but with some slight reservation. He may have heard the old saying about no house being big enough for two women.

Sometimes we put out "life-changing" suggestions to others, especially because we want to do the right thing, but do not really believe that our offer will be accepted. Together we decided that it really was the right time and the right thing to do. I do not think that Ray believed that his mother would accept this offer. As for me, I thought it would be more like when we had asked my dad to come with us. It took many invitations before he agreed. I thought it would take many offers before Charlotte would agree to come and live with us. To our surprise, this very independent, extremely private woman said yes to our first offer. We moved Charlotte into our home on a warm, sunny day in the summer of 1995.

One anecdote that has been retold many times about that day goes something like this. Our sons, JR and Matthew and a friend of JR's were helping with the move and had arrived with Grandmom's STUFF. The friend asked where we wanted him to put her shoes. I quickly replied, "Please, put them under the pool table in the basement." He looked at me with a questioning face and softly mused to himself, "Lady, you'll need at least three pool tables to accommodate all of her shoes." We all laughed and continued the procession of bringing in her STUFF: fourteen bathrobes, at least twelve umbrellas in every color under the sun, enough jewelry, belts and scarves to fill ten large plastic trash bags, dress slacks in stacks of a dozen of each color—the list could go on—and on— and on.

In hindsight, all of us were just too busy with our own lives to analyze this situation and put some thought into how absurd it was for Charlotte to have all of this STUFF. Charlotte gave JR and Karen a dining room set, coo-coo clock, chairs and other large household items, which at least solved the big furniture problems that could have occurred. Moving day was a good day for Charlotte. She invited her friend,

Mrs. Rose, to visit and seemed very happy and content with the move, and wanted to show off her new residence. I was proud of Ray and me that we could ease some of Charlotte's worries and be of help to her, imagining that my mom would be smiling down on me for doing the right thing.

# ♥ *Chapter Three...*

## *Charlotte Comes To Live with Us.*
*"...when someone comes for a visit,*
*it is much easier to be polite. However,*
*when they live with you, a dynamic is created*
*that makes it very difficult to ignore*
*the person or their issues."*
*Years 1995-2000*


Charlotte continued working as a hostess in one of the fast food chains and loved it. She kept to herself when she was home. She loved her privacy, and we tried to provide her with that. We invited her to have dinner with us every evening. Sometimes she would join us, but for the most part, she declined. We just chalked this up to her needing some adjustment time during this big change in her life.

We had times of concern when Charlotte first came to live with us that made us question how this was going to work. Matthew lives with us. One incident that I remember well involved him and his grandmother. After a day out, Matthew asked Charlotte how her day had been when she returned home. Charlotte looked him in the eye and said, "I don't have to answer to anybody about my comings and goings!" Matthew took all of this with a grain of salt as he tried to coax her into a conversation.

I reacted like a typical mother hen and told Charlotte that this was just what a family did when they came together at the end of a day. A family reconnects with talk of what happened during their day. I told her, in no uncertain terms, that it was unacceptable to speak to Matthew like that. I also said that I would be so happy if my adult grandson would be interested and kind enough to care about my day. It was hard for me to be so curt and blunt, but I did not want any more of this kind of dialogue in our home.

We were grateful that Charlotte had her license and her car to give her independence and autonomy. This kept us from having to plan schedules around her needs, so our life was not too disrupted by her living with us.

In retrospect, there were things to which we should have given more attention while Charlotte was still in her apartment. Some conversations with her about bizarre topics such as men with pink "stuff" on their mouths, people upstairs looking through the floor into her apartment and other such odd comments were passed off with a joking comment about her losing it. This kind of response let us off the hook, and we quickly went onto another subject.

Denial allows you to keep going on your own merry way. It pains me greatly to say that "out of sight, out of mind" was a truth that applied to Charlotte when she was on her own. Some of the odd things that were happening became more evident now that she lived under our roof.

More strange behaviors came to light, but deep within we still hosted denial. Ray and I would joke together with our sons and friends about how weird some of Charlotte's actions were, but we did not delve into them. I am truly sorry that I made fun or made quips about her or her actions. I feel embarrassed now because I did not show respect. Looking back, I said many things that were not considerate.

After a while, Ray and I noticed stacks of paper products piling up in the corners of her room; we were concerned that all this

17

could be a fire hazard. There were scads of used paper plates, napkins, coffee stirrers, cups, plastic spoons and forks. After asking her if she wanted help in cleaning up her room and getting a direct "No, nothing needs cleaning up or thrown away," we would go in every few days and remove some of the "coveted trash" when she was downstairs or out of the house. We found this trash gathering a bit crazy, but we just let it go. I guess we tried to avoid confrontation; we wanted Charlotte to feel welcome in what was now also her home.

Other examples of this kind of craziness surfaced. I began finding half-used toilet tissue and paper towel rolls in her room. All of us noticed that our silverware was disappearing and I finally decided to have a look in Charlotte's room. Of course, this was done while she was out. When I opened her dresser drawers, I was not prepared for what I found—half-eaten cookies, unopened pint-size cartons of milk, old pieces of fruit, dirty tissues—anything one might expect to find in a trash bag. Our missing silverware was also there! We chalked it up to Charlotte becoming eccentric and, for the most part, just kept up our secret clean-up procedure whenever she left the house. We would laugh at the four huge trash bags of garbage that we carried out on a weekly basis. I don't ever remember trying to put myself in Charlotte's shoes, so to speak.

Never did it occur to me that something medical was going on with her. Most likely, I did not want to face that possibility. If we consciously acknowledged that there was something medically wrong with Charlotte, Ray and I would be the ones who would have to handle her care.

To look at Charlotte, it would appear that not much had changed. But that was only if you did not get too close to her. Charlotte had always loved her perfume, but now she was wearing enough to gag those around her. When someone comes for a visit, it is much easier to be polite. However, when they live with you, a dynamic is created that makes it very difficult to ignore the person or her issues. I tried to talk to Charlotte about not using so much perfume, but that suggestion only offended her and made her go off in a huff. Charlotte never was one for confrontation of any kind, so walking away was a typical kind of behavior for her. I was between a rock and hard place in this situation.

Also, her body odor was telling us that she was not washing or bathing enough. So another secret mission began whenever she was out—taking a few of her clothes at a time and sending them to the cleaners or washing them myself and putting them back before she returned home.

This was a very trying time for Charlotte and for me. I always knew her to be so immaculate about her personal hygiene, and it was so distressing for me to know that others could be or would be offended by her body odor. I gently tried to offer new soaps and suggestions but was met with hostility. I knew that I would be hurt if someone told me that I had a personal hygiene problem. How would I react if my daughter-in-law said something like that to me? I felt like an intruder in someone's private space, like opening the bathroom door when occupied. It was uncomfortable, embarrassing and difficult to handle.

We did the best that we could with the situation and tried to just tolerate what was going on—or rather what was not going on—without alienating Charlotte. One of the most fascinating things that happens in dealing with parents' aging is how much you push aside and disregard—how much you choose not to acknowledge what you are experiencing. We, as loyal children, join our parent(s) in this not-so-gentle subterfuge.

Even when confrontations became more frequent, no bells or sirens went off in our minds. As previously mentioned, her usual method of handling conflict was to retreat and remove herself by walking away. She often took to passive-aggressive behavior, not speaking to us and sticking to the silent treatment for very long periods of time. Now we realize that when she started to become verbally combative, we should have paid more attention.

By 1999, we were seeing other things that concerned us about Charlotte such as ice cream containers left in the microwave, dirty underwear put back into dresser drawers, leaving the bathroom without turning off the water in the sink or not flushing the toilet. The parade of taking bags out to her car whenever she was going somewhere was another disturbing signal. Sometimes she would make seven or eight trips up and down the stairs from her room to her car, filling her trunk with these trash bags. When any one of us asked if she needed help, she would say that she was fine.

Upon arriving home, she repeated this same ritual, coming and going day after day. It was exhausting just watching her in this driven physical undertaking.

At this time, Ray started to find beer bottles in her trash and alerted me. Charlotte had never been a drinker. She might have a bottle of beer with seafood, but not anything close to the amount she must have been consuming each evening. Another sign missed. How mind boggling it is now to see clearly so many things that screamed out to us but did not get our attention!

Charlotte made very few remarks to us about having any difficulty with people at work. She loved her job and the people appreciated her hard work ethic; her job was her salvation. Charlotte never told us that her job was terminated or that she quit. We never found out what had happened. Charlotte just stopped going to work.

# ♥ Chapter Four...

## The Accident and Our Awakening
*"For us, denial was a welcomed way of dealing with things when we did not know what else to do or we did not want to deal with it."*
*Year 2001*

As for Charlotte's driving, we were concerned, and sometimes we would follow her in our car. For the most part, she did pretty well on our country roads except for traveling under the speed limit. We said a prayer each time she left and held our breath until she returned, but we had no control over her driving or not driving. She had a valid driver's license and drive she did—everyday!

In 2001, Charlotte had a minor accident on the main street in our little town. Ray, who was at work, received a call from the police officer at the scene informing him of the accident. He said that everyone was okay but stated that Charlotte was very confused.

Ray went to the accident scene and found his mother adamant about the other people hitting her car. She was insulted because the police officer had run over her foot. The officer cited her and recommended that she be retested in order to maintain a valid driver's license.

She was very upset and seemed to understand very little of what transpired. She could only focus on the audacity of that policeman to question her driving ability. It seemed like World War III had begun as she became very angry with Ray for allowing all of this to happen. She could not and would not accept that she would have to be retested in order to get a renewed license.

This situation was difficult for everyone. Knowing the independence driving gave Charlotte, yet being very aware that driving a car was not safe, either for her or for others, created a dilemma familiar to many families. The law took this privilege away from Charlotte. However, our family suffered her fury. In hindsight, we have called this our "awakening."

More of this awakening came the week following her accident when a man knocked on our door and served Charlotte with three summonses for unpaid credit card bills. She had been receiving many phone calls and very often would just hang up the phone in a huff. Evidently, she was receiving calls about her non-payment from collection agencies.

I noticed that when Charlotte talked with her friend on the phone, she did not seem to hear what Mrs. Rose was saying. Charlotte would talk non-stop and not listen to whatever was being said on the other end. Then Mrs. Rose called us one day to say that she and Charlotte had a falling out and that she just did not understand how all of it came about. She was upset and worried about her friend.

Ray and I both tried to talk to Charlotte about this situation but got nowhere. I even tried to listen as she spoke to herself endlessly about Mrs. Rose and what had happened. Charlotte would go through the same scenario repeatedly about her driving all the way to see Mrs. Rose and how she had been taken advantage of. Charlotte did this while rocking in her bedroom chair and she would bang the arm of her chair at the same exact sentence in her rhetoric. This, of course, was her version of the story, and she held on tightly to her anger. This could go on for hours at a time.

What could you do with someone so self-focused and consumed by her anger? I walked away frustrated, unwilling to give this situation any more of my time or energy.

It was after Charlotte's accident and those three summonses that Ray and I became much more aggressive in our involvement with Charlotte's affairs. We asked to help with her checkbook; reluctantly she gave it to us. We could not believe our eyes. There were checks half written out with dates in the amount line, made out incorrectly. It was a mess!

Then we went through more of her things and looked into those infamous "go-with-her-everywhere" trash bags. We found more check books in disarray. Credit card statements, bank statements, other important papers and every bit of jewelry she owned were in those trash bags. She was carrying everything precious to her with her. She was paranoid about those bags. She put them by the side of her bed and under her bed every night and took them with her whenever she left.

While all of this was going on, I had been in touch with our county's department on aging and was given the name of a geriatric specialist who could give Charlotte some testing. This wonderful woman came to our home and spent at least two hours with Charlotte. As I observed the testing, I was amazed at just how much of a deficit Charlotte had. It was difficult for her to understand the most simple of queries. I saw how cognitively challenged she was becoming. The doctor gave me the results of the evaluation. The diagnosis was that Charlotte was suffering from dementia and depression. She talked about the need for Charlotte to be in a senior's program that would get her out of house and around other people. She suggested the fine senior facilities that we have in our county and told us that she would be back for a follow-up visit. There was talk of a geriatric psychiatrist, but I did not give that the credence it deserved. In the beginning of this journey, I did not get the connection between what was going on with Charlotte's behaviors and the possibility of a mental health issue.

After Charlotte stopped driving, her life and our lives, with mutual space left for each of us, ceased to exist. We were responsible for all of her transportation needs. We lived in a part of the county with no public bus services. We would have to provide all of her transportation needs.

In trying to alleviate some of the pressure and isolation we were all feeling, we took the doctor's advice and made arrangements for Charlotte to attend a wonderful senior center and took Charlotte there two or three days a week. Eventually, we even arranged with a transportation service, Senior Bus Rides, to come to pick her up and bring her back home. This was a real break for us.

Charlotte was not thrilled with this good news. She was reluctant; she seemed hesitant to try something new. It took some convincing to get her to go to the center. However, after the first couple of days, she decided that it was a good thing. Her complaint about not being able to do anything now that she could no longer drive could be put to rest. She would be able to enjoy all that this center offered. Charlotte became very happy and excited about going to the center. She only missed going because of sickness. She really enjoyed the people, music and the activities. This was a great blessing for Charlotte and for us.

Things went along pretty well for a while, with the exception of her still blaming Ray for taking away her license. We were well aware of how important losing the privilege to drive was to Charlotte, but we could not seem to get this very angry woman to understand that we had not initiated her license loss. She constantly fussed, fumed and yelled at us about not being able to drive and not being able to be "on the go." We did not know how to handle her frequent outbursts. It was hard for us not to rationalize that, after all, she was going out three days a week to the senior center and loving every minute of it. I felt unappreciated for all of my efforts to keep Charlotte on the go and involved in great activities.

My dad went through this same crisis of losing his license but did not react like Charlotte. He just made statements like, "I really miss my car!" I realized that it was not fair to compare the two reactions, as two people can react very differently to the same situation. Still, I could not help thinking that it would have made it so much easier if Charlotte would have been more cooperative, more accepting.

Charlotte rode the bus to the senior center two or three times a week; we settled into this routine with optimistic relief. Ray and I took over her other travel needs and wrote the checks for her bills. The little bit of money she did have in the bank had been used to pay off her credit card debts.

The creditors stopped calling, but new credit cards were sent to her in the mail. How could a person in this state of financial crisis be offered more credit cards? It is, plain and simple, immoral behavior on the part of the credit companies and should be made a criminal offense!

In the meantime, Ray and I took Charlotte to see her primary care physician who had been her doctor for over twenty years. We saw first hand the rapport he had with her. They joked with one another just like old friends until the topic of her driving came up. He told us that he had been telling her for sometime that she should consider not driving anymore and that he was glad that this would now be the case. She was furious and turned on him just as she had turned on us. Charlotte's "Doctor Jekyll and Mr. Hyde" turnabout happened at that very moment.

The doctor who had come to our home to do the testing came back a month or so later and saw that Charlotte was doing better and attributed it to the fact that she was getting so much interaction and stimulation at the senior center. This was true as her days were filled with all of the activities the center offered and she was not spending so much time by herself. The doctor again mentioned that Charlotte should see a geriatric psychiatrist, but since her attitude was improving, I just dropped that piece of advice.

In hindsight, I wish that I had not let that valuable information go without further investigation and action. We did not see the importance of adding another layer of care.

Keeping things the same is easier and requires less energy and I certainly fell into that trap. Ray and I decided that since Charlotte had just gone through so many changes, we would stick with her regular doctor even though his office was a good distance from our home. We believed our concern for familiarity was the right decision.

The senior center that Charlotte attended at that time was very large, socially active and a model for many other facilities. About a year after she had started attending the center, I received a call from the staff director who told me that Charlotte did not seem to be able to fit in anymore. She was acting anxious, following the leaders around with non-stop questions about what was coming next and what she should be doing. The woman told me that it may be time for Charlotte to attend another center more equipped to handle Charlotte's changing behaviors. I kept telling the woman that Charlotte loved the senior center and really enjoyed playing bingo and participating in the music program. I thanked her for her concern but left it at that. After two more calls, the leader at the center had to be blunt with me. She told me that if I kept sending Charlotte to the senior center, she would have to get in touch with "the authorities." I was told that there were incidents of people dropping off their elderly family member and using the center as an adult day care facility. The implication was clear that we could be one of those families.

By now, Ray and I were so steeped in denial about how truly changed Charlotte's behavior was becoming that, in retrospect, such strong words were necessary for me to open my eyes and see what was happening without my rose colored glasses. I now asked, "Where could Charlotte go?" The staff told me of an adult day care center in the same complex that would be appropriate for Charlotte. I called and made an appointment to see the facility and signed Charlotte up the very next day. She would attend two days a week. There was a snag, however. Their bus did not come out this far into the county, so

I would take her in the morning and Ray would pick her up in the afternoon.

There was another center in the western part of our county that was a more secure facility where Charlotte could attend. We arranged for her to go there the other three days a week. This center had bus service, and this was a great help to us. The only drawback was that there was a broad timetable for when the bus would arrive to pick her up and when it would drop her off. She had to be ready by 8:00 a.m., but sometimes the bus did not pick her up until after 9:00 a.m. The same thing happened in the afternoon in that she could be dropped off anywhere from 12:30 p.m. to 3:30 p.m. depending on what programs they had that day. I had to be ever mindful of being home by 12:30 pm. as someone had to be home to get Charlotte from the bus. My life was being ruled by a bus schedule on those three days.

We were in such denial as to what all of Charlotte's bizarre behavior might indicate. Why? For us, denial was a welcomed way of dealing with things when we did not know what else to do or we did not want to deal with it. We had been telling ourselves that Charlotte was just getting older, and we used the term "eccentric" to describe Charlotte. Yes, Charlotte was repeating herself, telling us the same thing over and over. Wasn't that a common thing in the elderly? Forgetting things and short-term memory loss are signs of getting older along with some other "quirky" behaviors. Is that not so?

This part of our journey with all of the responsibility of making Charlotte's doctor appointments, finding new senior centers for her to attend, as well as lining up the transportation and taking over her finances was hectic. We were trying to do the very best that we could for Charlotte with each one of our decisions. There were several visits with Charlotte's primary care physician. He confirmed the dementia and depression diagnosis of the geriatric doctor. These doctors said many things to us. There is indeed proof in the statement, that we retain only one out of ten spoken statements. I may not remember which doctor said it first, but I will never forget the words, "Charlotte has Alzheimer's!"

# ♥ *Chapter Five...*

*Charlotte has Alzheimer's!*
*"Okay, now Charlotte was diagnosed.*
*What would it mean for her and for us?*
*We had no idea."*
*Fall 2001*


Charlotte has Alzheimer's disease.

She has Alzheimer's.

Charlotte has Alzheimer's!

I had heard of that term before. We even had friends that had said their parent(s) had been diagnosed with Alzheimer's. Ray's Aunt Ann, Charlotte's sister-in-law, died a few years ago and she had Alzheimer's, but we were not in close contact with that part of our family anymore, so we did not know very much about their story. Okay, now Charlotte was diagnosed. What would it mean for her and for us? We had no idea. We could not have imagined how this dreadful disease would consume our lives. Alzheimer's—the newest diagnosis on the block for the elderly.

When Ray and I first began to talk about his mother having Alzheimer's, we did not know what to say to one another. We just looked at each other, our minds racing, but not really knowing exactly where to begin. Ray absorbs new events in a very logical, thoughtful way and needs time to reflect. I did my usual thing—react. I went through the papers the doctor had given me and went on the web to see what information I could gather. Day after day, I looked for more information.

*The Alzheimer's Association succinctly defines Alzheimer's disease (AD) as a "progressive, neurodegenerative disease characterized by loss of function and death of nerve cells in several areas of the brain, leading to loss of mental functions such as memory and learning." The American Psychiatric Association's more elaborate definition for "dementia of the Alzheimer's type" speaks of "multiple cognitive deficits," with gradual onset and continuing decline from a person's prior level of functioning (American Psychiatric Association 1994, at 142). As a recent review article summarizes,*

*"The clinical hallmarks are progressive impairment in memory, judgment, decision making, orientation to physical surrounding, and language" (Nussbaum and Ellis 2003). Neuropsychiatric symptoms, such as agitation, depression, and delusions are also common in AD patients (Mega, Masterman, O'Connor et al, 1999)* [1-1]

*Dementia is a disorder characterized by multiple impairments of cognition in an individual who is otherwise fully alert and attentive. The impairments of intellectual functioning include memory, abstraction, judgment, and language (Rabins 2001). Although at least 75 distinct diseases can present as a dementia syndrome, Alzheimer's disease is the most common type of progressive dementia, accounting for around two-thirds of dementia cases (Cummings and Cole 2002; Mace and Rabins 1999, at 290; Nussbaum and Ellis 2003; Post 1998; Rabins 2001).* [1-2]

Having Charlotte diagnosed with Alzheimer's was just that, a diagnosis. We were told that she was in the first or mildest stage of the disease, which is characterized predominately by memory impairment. This diagnosis at least put a name to and a body of reason for the unexplained behaviors we had been witnessing over the past six or seven years.

I started to read and investigate everywhere—on the web, in books and at the department on aging—to obtain any and all information about Alzheimer's. If any blurb came on the television about Alzheimer's, I would stop dead in my tracks and listen for details. I watched every show that came on that had any thing to do with the illness. If anyone mentioned the word "Alzheimer's," my ears would perk up; I was like a hungry animal picking up the needed sounds to guide me to my prey.

Charlotte continued with the hoarding of things—things of value and things that were worthless. I learned by trial and error how to handle this situation better. I stopped confronting her about these kinds of behaviors. This prevented much turmoil and tension between us. I just kept getting rid of trash when she was not around. Most of the time, her short-term memory loss kept her from remembering what she had actually accumulated.

Now that we had a diagnosis, I wish that I could say that I found her behaviors easier to deal with, but I did not, at least not all of them. The bathing issue was still a real source of contention. I even got to the point of warning her that if she did not wash herself properly, I would do it for her. That did not go over well. Charlotte's non-verbal body language spoke volumes to me. She pulled her robe tightly around her and gave me a look that could kill. She stomped off and slammed her bedroom door in my face. There I stood, wondering, "What good was it to put clean clothes on a dirty, smelly body?" Normal logic was mine, not Charlotte's. I have since learned that the ability to smell is the first of the senses lost by an Alzheimer's patient. Things certainly do become clearer in hindsight!

One morning, I made the decision that this situation was getting out of hand and her health could be jeopardized by her lack of personal cleanliness. I had to get over my self-consciousness and do what needed to be done. I just began to help her get undressed. Placing a warm, large robe around her and without any mention of what I was actually going to do next, led her into the shower. I kept making small, happy talk about her being a beautiful woman and talked about her jewelry. Before I knew it, she was in the shower telling me how good it felt. I just gave her the washcloth and let her wash herself any way she chose. Just having the water running on her was a good omen. I washed her hair. It had been so long since we had even seen Charlotte's own hair. She covered it up with wigs.

When she first started wearing wigs, she chose beautiful and complimentary ones. As the years, passed, the wigs became matted and disheveled; she no longer had them washed and set and the wigs just added to the untidiness of her appearance. The wig was off and finally I got her hair washed!

Now she was clean from head to toe. My constant attempts to keep her modest with her robe and towels and not talking about taking the shower had paid off. In this case, action did work better than words. As the water in the shower swirled out, I remember feeling so drained, as if I, too, were emotionally going down that drain. Unconsciously, I must have had some awareness that now I had initiated another caretaking solution that I would be responsible for on a regular basis. I sensed that more of my freedom was spiraling down with the water and being taken away, even though at the time I did not dare put this into a conscious thought. After that first shower, it became at least a tri-weekly ritual for the two of us.

I removed the wigs from Charlotte's room. Whenever she asked about them, I told her that they were being washed, hoping that if the wigs were out of her sight, she would eventually forget about them. Sadly, yet mercifully, she did forget about them.

One observation I made from the bathing experience was that touching is so important. I always felt Charlotte's body relax when rubbing lotion on her back or legs. Combing her hair and fixing it for her was so soothing that she often closed her eyes and drifted off to another space in her mind. A slight smile would turn her grimaced face into a "this feels good" portrait.

I even found myself a bit more relaxed and felt happy that I was offering Charlotte this kind of peacefulness. While she did not actually say "thank you," her reaction let me know that my effort was well received. This connection for Charlotte and me was not accomplished very often, but in the bathing and hair fixing, we often had our closest times.

In early winter of 2001, my sister, Be, was in a nursing home dying from lung cancer. We knew that she did not want to die in a hospital setting. She asked if we would bring her home with us. We did so and made arrangements for her hospice care for the two weeks before she died and on her way to heaven. She would ask me to give her back rubs and always told me how wonderful a back rub was.

Touch makes a connection; it conveys caring. It says that you want to make things a little bit better. Touching with a gentle, easy motion gives some sense of rejuvenation and can be a way of offering pleasure to any one suffering.

# ♥ Chapter Six...

## Living with Alzheimer's

*"'You hate me and I hate you!'*
*This was not true, but she would*
*fixate on these kinds of statements."*

With the pack rat and bathing issues pretty well under control, Charlotte and I had less tension between us. It was not until she became very critical of Ray that things began to become stressful again on a regular basis. She would say the most hurtful things to him or about him. Charlotte started by saying things such as Ray never liked her or loved her. She would say that he did not want her with us anymore. Charlotte would look him in the eye and shout, "You hate me and I hate you!" This was not true, but she would fixate on these kinds of statements.

At times, just Ray's presence would ignite the flame of her fiery words, and it was better if he just left the room. I felt tortured; like my heart was being ripped out as I watched Ray's face when her words cut into him. Ray knew that his mother did not mean those horrible things, but that did not keep him from feeling terrible when those words were screamed at him.

I could not understand or accept those harsh, cruel remarks about her only child, a very fine man in whom she should have been so proud. It was a pain that I wanted to erase for him. He did not deserve this kind of lashing. It was not easy to overlook or smooth over. Even though this was coming from the illness, it was one of the hardest things to take. It would send chills down my spine, and I would shudder at her lack of control. My clenched teeth would bite down so hard that my jaw would rebel with "enough already!" How could a mother speak to her own child this way?

I did have someone tell me that the person who is loved the most is the one who gets the most abuse. Ray was the point man for Charlotte's assults, and it was, for me, the saddest thing to witness in the entire struggle.

By the end of 2001, Charlotte became obsessed and paranoid about people coming into her room "stealing things." She did not even want our granddaughters, who were then five and six years old, upstairs when she was downstairs. She trusted no one.

She once accused a man who was installing carpet upstairs of going into her room and taking her things. I was mortified, red-faced as I asked the man to forgive her and to, please, understand that it was her illness acting out. Yes, it was the illness, my head knew that, but my calm outside reaction that others saw was very often so different on the inside. Inside I would be screaming at Charlotte's behavior. I expected her to be better behaved. I was frustrated and humiliated. It was as if dark heavy robes were on my shoulders, and I just wanted to be able to shake them off. I was embarrassed and frustrated by Charlotte's outbursts.

It is much easier in our society to accept physical disease than it is to accept mental disease. Our American culture just seems to like well-behaved human beings at any age and assigns nobility to suffering in good humor, or maybe that is how I see it and believe that everyone else sees it the same way.

Many times, after handling one of Charlotte's episodes, I became remorseful and very critical of myself. Guilt would engulf me, as I would remember the very different circumstances when taking care of my dad. I did not remember ever losing my cool with him. I knew that as he aged, his body was failing him but Daddy's mind was still sharp. It was so much easier to care for him.

I recall that while caring for Daddy, my prayers always included a petition for good health as I grow old. I did not give a thought to how this petition, focused on good health, would soon come to have a different slant.

My morning ritual with Charlotte consisted of laying out her clothes, making sure that she washed herself and brushed her teeth. She always combed her hair, put on her lipstick and never failed to put on her jewelry. I had become the keeper of her perfume and would monitor how much she put on to keep the fragrance from being overpowering.

After her personal needs were seen to, Charlotte watched me as I put her treasured trash bags into her closet and would close her bedroom door behind us before we went downstairs. Then I would fix her breakfast and wait with her for the bus or get her into the car and take her to the adult day care center.

Ray would pick her up after work, and she would want to retreat to her room and do her own thing. To be honest, I was glad she chose to stay in her own room. Then we did not have to listen to her complaints.

Back in her room, she was making sure that all of her possessions were still there; this took hours of pulling everything out and putting it back. Charlotte was still content to keep to herself with soft mutterings of discontent about one thing or another.

It was around this time that I had my first experience with Charlotte getting a urinary tract infection (UTI). Let me say unequivocally that urinary tract infections in someone suffering with dementia can be explosive. One evening Charlotte went to bed and we kept hearing noises from her room. I went in to check on her periodically, and she just seemed very restless. As the night wore on, she became physically unable to stop moving around in her bed. She did not indicate that anything was hurting or bothering her. However, her body never stopped moving that night as she tossed turned and raised her legs and arms up into the air. Ray and I sat with her that long, long night until morning; she never slept. I called her doctor in the morning and he immediately stated that Charlotte probably had a urinary tract infection and sent medicine out for her. He was right, she was able to sleep the following night.

This episode taught me a valuable lesson about UTIs and the way a patient with dementia reacts to having this kind of infection; I became ever watchful for these kinds of symptoms. UTI was the first thing I had checked out when Charlotte's behavior became uncontrollable, erratic or aggressive.

Sleep issues were becoming a major concern for Charlotte. She was not sleeping very well. She would go to sleep quickly enough but wake up in the middle of the night and begin to pull things out of her closet and dresser drawers.

Sometimes she was quiet; then there were times when she fussed and fumed about something she considered amiss. I would awaken and realize that she was downstairs. I would go down only to find her confused, and agitated.

After a visit to the doctor revealed that Charlotte's changing behaviors meant that more deterioration had taken place, he told us that, for her safety, we should lock her bedroom door at night. I could not do that. We would have to reverse the lock to the outside of the door in order to keep her locked in and that seemed cruel to me. She would be unable to see out. She would not have access to her bathroom. We would have to find another solution to Charlotte's roaming.

Several store-bought baby gates for the hallway were tried but Charlotte knocked them down. Since we were very concerned for her safety on the stairs, Ray built an open wooden gate that he put across the hallway. We tied it shut at bedtime with a beautiful wide ribbon. Charlotte cut it and went downstairs. Ray used a thick cord and the same thing happened. Charlotte just kept finding ways to be "free"—fulfilling the human spirit's desire for freedom.

We had gone through Charlotte's room with a fine-tooth comb and removed any thing that could be unsafe or dangerous for her to have in her possession. How she kept finding scissors and such things just boggled my mind. She was always finding hidden treasures that only God knew from where they came. Finally, a small metal chain and lock was used to secure the gate. Charlotte was able to move freely between her bedroom, the guest room and her bathroom if she woke up. The gate kept her away from the steps. This worked fine for about three or four months until we found her trying to open one of the guest room windows in the middle of the night. Since the bedrooms were on the second floor this frightened us and the gate was put in a new position, allowing her access only to her room and the bathroom.

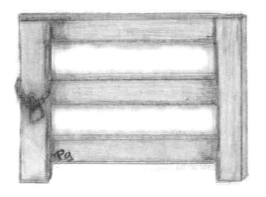

*"The Gate"*

I hated that locked gate. It would often enter my mind, "How would I be if locked behind a gate?" It was so difficult to accept this means of keeping her from harm. My mind knew it was for her safety, but that did not make it an easy thing to do.

At this point, Charlotte was able to realize, for the most part, that the gate was necessary to keep her from going down the steps by herself at night. She would admit to being afraid of falling, and we also shared that concern. The gate worked great, and it gave us peace of mind and allowed us to sleep somewhat more restfully.

Charlotte's knees and shoulders became arthritic over the years. Her knees especially gave her much pain. Getting up from a sitting position, she often had to wait to get her balance. She was really a good sport about this, often making a quip about "the ole gray mare ain't what she used to be!" I was, and still am, touched by her drive to keep on going and not give in to the pain.

The thirteen steps that she had to go down to the first floor were of great concern to me, as she had a few stumbles but, thank God, she caught herself without a serious fall. Being very cautious after those mishaps, Charlotte always went down the steps with me in front of her. She would place one hand on the railing and one hand on my shoulder as I held onto the railing with both of my hands for more stability. This worked beautifully, and we did this every trip down. At one point after Charlotte had been sick for a few days, I insisted that she go down "the rump-bump way," which was one step at a time on her bottom. I was not sure how steady she was, so going down this way gave us both some peace of mind.

When Charlotte was ascending the steps, I would go behind her, placing my hand on the small of her back, giving her a little more support to keep her from falling backward. Also, I sometimes would grab hold of her belt or the waistband of her slacks and give a little tug to help her lift up her feet to the next step. This made those thirteen steps a bit easier for her to ascend.

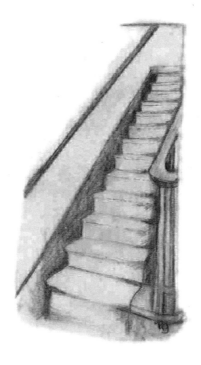

*"The Thirteen Steps"*

I was always looking for ways to keep Charlotte from getting hurt. Then came the day when I "saved" Charlotte's life. It was after we had started our bathing ritual. Charlotte was showered in our bathroom because there was a seat in it so she could sit down. I usually fixed her hair there, but this time we went back into her bedroom as Ray was ready to get his shower. Charlotte was talking as I set her hair. I had put on her bra and had the terrycloth robe down around her waist covering her up. I noticed that she seemed to want to go backward and I chided her to sit up, stating that she could take a nap when we were finished. With those words out of my mouth, Charlotte fell back on the bed; her eyes rolled back into her head and she went limp. "Oh, dear God, please, please help me," I pleaded, as she began to have some sort of seizure.

Charlotte had an ashen color and could not be aroused. My body shook all over; my hands trembled and I kept repeating, "You are not going to die on me," as I called out for Ray or Matthew, but to no avail; they were not within earshot. I had to do something, and for some unknown reason, my mind was only thinking of getting her body to the side. I tried to lift her and move her, but her weight was too much for me. I grabbed the arms of her bathrobe and used them to roll her over. Still nothing—there were no signs of Charlotte coming around.

Getting her head lower than her body was my next goal, and again, with the robe as a sling, I pulled and tugged her off of the bed, head first. As soon as her head was lower than her abdomen, Charlotte started to cough. I stood in front of her and folded her down off the bed onto the floor.

She was choking and threw up a bit; my calls for help were finally heard downstairs, and Ray called 911. The paramedics came and when the events were recanted, one of the medics told me that I had done all of the right things. Amid the shaking and nervousness, I felt so relieved to have her breathing and talking. The paramedics checked all of her vitals and found everything okay but were not able to offer a definite answer as to what caused Charlotte to lose consciousness.

When leaving, the same paramedic turned to me and said, "Ma'am, you saved your mother-in-law's life!" I did not know how to respond.

# ♥ Chapter Seven...

## Help

*"I now know that, as with a child,
it does indeed 'take a village' to care
for the Alzheimer patient."*
Year 2002

Two main resources made it possible for us to keep Charlotte with us—the adult day care centers and respite care.

Respite care is offered by some adult day care centers, assisted-living facilities or assisted-living houses. In our county, we are "rich" in assisted-living houses, which are converted private homes that are equipped to handle the elderly in small numbers. Most of the residences take "live-in" elders who are unable to be on their own anymore, and for a wide range of reasons, do not live with their families. Some offer respite care for families needing care for their loved one while they are away. It is not a permanent stay, just for a specified amount of time. The Department on Aging is a resource for getting this kind of information on the assisted-living private homes in any given area.

Some words of caution are necessary. Not all places, whether they are adult day care centers, large assisted-living facilities or the smaller assisted-living houses, are equal. The state and the county regulate all these facilities, but it takes a lot of legwork and investigation to find the good ones. It is the only way that I could ever leave Charlotte in someone else's care. The time and effort paid off because we left Charlotte in good hands and always returned to find her content and well.

We used respite care for vacation time or when I had the chance to go with Ray on a business trip. Sometimes we took advantage of respite if we were going to have a gathering of some kind or had a week filled with activities. Respite care always provided a well-needed reprieve for Ray and for me. Ray and I both enjoyed having our time to ourselves, even if it was only for a short time. At times though, when we were having family gatherings and judged they would be too much for Charlotte to handle, I felt guilty. I struggled because I did not want Charlotte to be left out—inclusion is so important to me. But at the same time, I was relieved to be away from Charlotte.

The adult day care center offered respite care, and I found two other assisted-living houses that also offered this service. Ray and I will always be indebted to Yolanda for the wonderful care she gave to Charlotte in our absence. Yolanda took such good care of Ray's mom. She kept her immaculate.

When we would pick Charlotte up, the two of them would be laughing, or if they were in a testy situation, Yolanda would be doing her very best to get Charlotte back into a better frame of mind. When Charlotte was with Yolanda, I was confident that Charlotte was taken care of just as I took care of her. This was a great source of comfort for me.

Charlotte was not able to stay by herself anymore, so we appreciated that we were fortunate to have Matthew around to stay with her some evenings while we went out. Whenever we asked, Matthew would try and accommodate our request. Matthew was very good to his grandmother.

My sister, Jean, was a god-send to us. She was available at times to keep Ray's mom with her if something came up during the early evening hours. At first, it was very difficult for me to ask and then to accept her kind offers of help. I now know that, as with a child, it does indeed "take a village" to care for the Alzheimer patient.

It is a critical part of survival! It was a critical part of our survival to accept help when offered and to ask for help when needed. This deserves to be repeated. It is critical to accept help when it is offered and to ask for help when it is needed. Sometimes, your request for help may be putting out someone else, but it still is necessary that the caregiver ask for help and respite.

All caregivers must realize that when someone offers help, if you cannot think of something specific for them to do, let them come to sit, talk and listen to you or let them sit with the Alzheimer's patient. You then can take a long soak in the bathtub or a refreshing shower with the peace of mind that someone else is on guard.

Many churches have "Good Samaritan" groups, and often a neighbor might be able to offer you a little break from the Alzheimer's patient's demands. Also, many senior centers have support groups. Take advantage of what they have to offer. Help comes in many forms. We could not have cared for Charlotte without the help from others.

Help was even present in four-footed friends. Our Matthew's dog, Marley, was a great source of amusement for Charlotte.

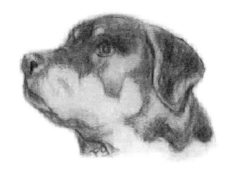

*Marley—Charlotte's "great-granddog"*

At one time, Charlotte had hated the dog and was frightened of her. Marley is a one-hundred-pound Rottweiller with the mind set of a big timid oaf. Since her illness,

"Marley-girl" and Charlotte have spent hours just sitting together with Charlotte petting the dog and fussing over her.

Who could know? We became very grateful for the time that Marley amused Charlotte and kept her content.

Helpful ideas also give the assistance that is needed at times to deal with the Alzheimer's patient. Having an open mind when others offer suggestions is such a necessary element for learning.

I remember when one of the center's staff suggested that Charlotte wear an apron. At first, I did not get the point of why she should do this. Then as we talked more about it, I could see that she could put her "picked-up-treasures" into the apron pockets and not stuff them down in the legs of her slacks. She often did this when she wore pants with no pockets. When her clothes were taken off, I often found pieces of sandwiches, rubber gloves, artificial flowers and many other coveted items.

Now, Charlotte stuffed those apron pockets full and all that had to be done was to take the apron off her. She did not get that we were taking her "valuables" away from her. She wore the apron every day. It was a great idea.

As Charlotte slipped deeper into the jaws of Alzheimer's, her obsessive needs were focused on wanting to go out all the time. By evening, she did not remember being out during the day at the center and wanted to know when she was going out. When she looked around our family room and observed that only Ray and I were there, she believed that "everyone else" had gone out, and we were keeping her at home and not letting her go, too.

Charlotte would also fuss that she never got anything to eat or drink. She would become agitated and unmanageable, especially in the early evening. She would throw anything that she was holding and bang on her chair. She became a real handful!

I found that a lollipop given to Charlotte at the first signs of this kind of agitation did the trick. For just about an hour she would "suck that pop" and be content and happy with the world.

Television for the most part confused and agitated Charlotte. If the news was on, she would think that the newscasters were harassing her personally. She would talk to the TV just as if the people on the screen were right there in the family room with her. She could no longer distinguish what was happening to her from what was happening around her. If she saw something like a fire or disaster, it consumed her thoughts. She actually believed that her life was in danger or that the police were after her. We finally had to give up watching that kind of TV.

Charlotte loved watching the animal shows. That was good except that the commercials sometime upset her, so Ray just taped the episodes without commercials and filled a tape for her to watch. Charlotte would belly laugh at the animal antics. "Baby Einstein" tapes were good, too.

Just as my sister, Jean, and "Marley-girl" were a source of joy and comfort to Charlotte, so were our granddaughters, Kelsey and Kayla. They knew at mealtime or snack time that Great-Grandmom got her food first. It was such a tender sight to witness them catering to her and making sure that she was served before everyone else.

It was so touching to see the two little girls play with their great-grandmother. Charlotte would allow the girls to adorn her with their dress-up clothes. They would wrap bright colored, feathered boas and shawls around her and place large brimmed hats upon her head. It was a charming, tender sight and one I hold dear to my heart.

At the same time, I was pained by the fact that the little girls would eventually outgrow this kind of play but that Charlotte would only regress and keep becoming more childlike because of this disease. What a pitiful reality!

# ❤ *Chapter Eight...*

## *The Disease Keeps Progressing*

*"The staff at the Senior Center Plus had no choice but to tell us that she was no longer an appropriate candidate for their program."*

### *Years 2003-2004*

I should mention here that we knew that Charlotte had developed some "kleptomaniac" tendencies as the reality of what actually belonged to her and what did not had eroded. She was constantly picking up things that did not belong to her. Ray and I were continually returning a bag full of "swiped" articles from the center or the respite places. We were always welcomed with much understanding and gratefulness for returning what Charlotte had taken.

I remember when I found my watch on her arm. I thought I had lost it in the garden.

I informed her that she had my watch. She looked at me and stated unequivocally, "I am not a thief!" My heart actually skipped a beat at the sincerity and the truthfulness of her statement. She certainly was not a thief. What humiliation the Alzheimer patient suffers. Alzheimer's disease is the thief.

One day I received a call from the staff leader of the Senior Center Plus, telling me that Charlotte had a large sum of cash in her purse. I checked where I had kept money for vacation, and the money was missing. When Charlotte got home that day, I looked in her purse and sure enough, there was a "wad" of $20 bills. The staff at this center was so good to Charlotte. What a dedicated and sincere group of honest, caring women. I know this beyond a doubt.

The Senior Center Plus staff kept in communication with me while Charlotte attended their center. They asked if I had any tips on how to best handle certain difficult situations with Charlotte. I would tell them some of the things that I did to ease Charlotte's agitated temperament.

When she became irritated and grouchy, I would start fussing about her jewelry. That always seemed to work. If that didn't soothe her attitude and her negative behavior progressed, I would offer her a piece of candy as a distraction. That usually did the trick. The staff took my suggestions and it worked for them, too.

Behaviors that were more peculiar surfaced, and she was now making a constant noise in her throat. I would gently rub her neck to try to get her to stop, but for the most part, it was always there. It could be like a dripping faucet noise that just gets to you after awhile. I knew how annoying it could be and knew it could be bothering others as well. The doctor had no input as to how to curb this condition.

Early in 2003, the wonderful staff leader at the Senior Center Plus informed me that Charlotte needed "one on one" attention for which they were unequipped. They were dedicating one person to Charlotte, which was a real strain on their staffing needs.

When Charlotte became belligerent and started to use vulgar language and could not be redirected with any of our usual diversions, the staff at the Senior Center Plus had no choice but to tell us that she was no longer an appropriate candidate for their program. The staff said that she was their lowest functioning attendee, and although sympathetic, they had to request that Charlotte not attend anymore.

Hearing this from the caring staff pierced my heart. Oh, I knew it was true, but I did not want to hear it—another sign of things getting worse for Charlotte, for me and for us. I knew that they had allowed Charlotte to attend much longer than other centers may have. The entire staff gave Charlotte lots of special attention. I will always be so grateful for how kind and caring they were to Charlotte while she was there.

Again, we were fortunate in that the adult day care center which Charlotte was attending two days a week was able to take Charlotte for the three days that she had been attending at the Senior Center Plus. She would now attend only one facility, the adult day care center. This terrific center was staffed and equipped to better handle her declining mental challenges. The staff was good to Charlotte and so supportive to me. She liked all of the activities, especially the music, bingo and arts and crafts.

Having Charlotte leave the Senior Center Plus made what was actually happening clearer to me. It was difficult for me to see that she was slipping more into her own separate world.

Charlotte was now assessed as entering the middle stages of Alzheimer's. *(The second, middle or moderate stage of AD is described as additional impairments in language, the performance of everyday learned activities, recognition of the familiar and the "executive function" (the ability to initiate, sustain, and stop activities and to be mentally flexible) added to the memory impairment of the first or mild stage of AD.)*[1-3]

One aspect of Charlotte's behavior that increased greatly was how much she would ramble on and on in a soft-spoken voice about any number of every day topics: the flowers outside, her clothing, jewelry or Marley. If you listened closely, her conversations were understandable and cohesive but I could not converse with Charlotte about anything that she was saying. She was on "auto-pilot" with her own fast-track-speech-pattern, and she was incapable of adjusting the flow or taking in any conversation that I might try to make about what she was saying.

The same was true when she would go on and on about being beaten up when she got out of her car and how "they" had almost killed her. Charlotte had mentioned this to me months and months before when it was still possible to have a somewhat "give and take" conversation with her.

At that time, she implied that I knew about this terrible beating. Well, I had never heard about it, and I did not know if it really had happened to her or if she was mixed up and imagined that something like this had happened. She became infuriated when I told her that I knew nothing about anything like that happening to her. Charlotte became insistent that I did indeed know. At that time, I did not realize that the best policy is to go along with her and just say something like "I am so sorry that this happened to you." I tried to tell her that if this attack had occurred, she did not tell us about it. It was as if I were trying to talk a four-year old child out of believing in the tooth fairy or Santa Claus. Charlotte would not budge in her conviction. I wish I had known to accept what she was saying.

Today, I think that there was some truth to the episode she described. (Some experts say that the Alzheimer patient expresses present feelings of loneliness and fear by recounting some traumatic episodes like beatings or other traumatic experiences, but those things probably did not actually happen to them.) However, underneath the bizarre and odd behaviors, I believe that a deep part of the Alzheimer patient is alive and screaming from a place that we cannot get to from where we are. It is that authentic part of the person which cannot be heard and seen by the rest of us. It is so masked by those dismal symptoms.

Charlotte's bedtime routine became more time consuming and difficult. She hallucinated about "those people up there" while pointing to the tops of the curtain rods. "They" were coming down to get her, and she was going to beat the s___ out of them. Her behavior was little by little becoming more aggressive and harder to handle. At first, I tried to convince her that no one was there. That did not work at all. It was so real for her that nothing I could say would change what she believed. I just played along and sometimes would shoo her tormentors away and tell them not to come back if they knew what was good for them. I kept thinking that if anyone walked in, they would have us both committed. I felt self-conscious even though I was in my own home. I was uncomfortable but knew that I had to play the game. That approach to the imaginary demons worked most of the time. Turning Charlotte away from the windows and putting her on her side while rubbing her back calmed her on many nights.

At different times, night-lights created shadows that enlivened some of Charlotte's hallucinations, so I did away with them. At other times, a bright light was the answer to keeping her calmer. I just kept trying one thing or another until something worked.

I often wished that I was aware of a drug that could be given that would give her peace and me quiet. The doctor did try some sleep medications but none worked that well on a regular basis. He told me that, if over-medicated, Charlotte could more easily fall, and I did not want to happen. I see no benefit to taking drugs unless they do some good, so I discontinued giving them to her. I discussed this with Charlotte's doctor, and he agreed that there was no need to give her drugs that were not helping her.

By now, getting Charlotte to bed and having her stay in bed were constant challenges. It was about this time that I tried some different things at bedtime. Charlotte had always loved music, so Ray and I found songs from the forties and fifties and put them on a CD. In fact, our friend put them on an MP3 disk, which could play for twelve hours or so. Ray and I bought an inexpensive MP3 "boom box" and were all set.

There was a remote control for the music player that I could turn on or off from our bedroom. This worked great as Charlotte would lie in her bed, listen to the music and sing along. When she stopped singing with the music, I would hit the remote to turn off the player and not have to get out of bed.

Oh, how I wish that these good ideas had a longer life. The routine became one of constantly trying one solution and then another if that attempt did not succeed.

# ❤ Chapter Nine...

## Alzheimer's Takes More of Charlotte

*"Alzheimer's takes the golden threads of who you are and tangles them into a knotted mass ...that cannot be untangled."*

*Year 2004*

There was always a jolt of sadness each time something else had to be taken away from Charlotte. It was not a desire to keep taking things from her; it was just so necessary in order to keep her from harm. Her car taken because of no license, her freedom restricted because of the upstairs gate and now it was her earrings. It might not seem like much—earrings—but Charlotte loved them dearly. Her cherished earrings were now becoming a problem. Her ears were being mutilated as she had torn the earring holes trying to get several earrings into one hole. Finally, after finding her bleeding and confused, her pierced earrings had to go. I tried the clip-on kind, but they only lasted a little while, as she lost or misplaced them.

Most of Charlotte's good jewelry was put away for safekeeping, but she loved her costume jewelry, too. She had many lovely necklaces and often tried to wear every one of them at the same time. When I found her with them so tightly wound around her neck that she was actually strangling herself, it was apparent that these too would have to go. I put one on her each day, but truly it just wasn't the same for her.

Around this same time, when she did not sleep at night, she would quietly empty her entire closet onto her bed and put on as many articles of clothing as she could. I would go into her room and find her with three pairs of slacks on, two or three pairs of socks, the same number of sweaters and a coat or two to top off the ensemble.

I was not concerned about this behavior until one morning when I found her sweating and lethargic and was sure she must be dehydrated after being bundled up in so many articles of clothing. I was scared that I would find her in a heap, unconscious, from being overdressed. Therefore, a lock was put on her closet doors. She did not acknowledge or seem to mind the lock; if things were out of her sight, she usually did not seem to miss them.

One day after getting her dressed, I went into the guest room and got sidetracked with something there. All of a sudden I heard Charlotte exclaim with such jubilation, "Oh, look what I found!" Hurrying back into her room, I saw that her face was lit up like a Christmas tree, and her eyes sparkled as she reveled in her find. She kept saying, "I found a whole wardrobe—I found a whole wardrobe." She was ecstatic. (By this time, many of her clothes had been removed from her closet—what remained now was a mini-version of Charlotte's former wardrobe.)

I had forgotten to put the lock on the closet and when she was able to open those doors, she was beside herself with joy and delight.

Charlotte was a sharp dresser and had many beautiful outfits. She definitely was a "clothes hound" and loved each and every piece of clothing. In her state of mind, it may have been as if she had walked into a clothing store and found it filled with clothes she liked—imagine—all in her size! I could not help but rejoice right along with her. It was so touching, even though I knew that the closet had to be locked once again and the treasures inside kept from her. You can never be prepared for this kind of situation or the effect it can have on you.

Our emptying out her dresser, chest of drawers and her nightstands was another task that removed more of her belongings. Charlotte was losing more knowledge of the proper use for things. Finding her with an extension cord wrapped around her waist or neck, used as a belt or scarf, forced us to keep only a few books and other non-toxic belongings in her room.

She had dismantled all of the pictures and wall accessories and ruined most of them by stuffing them under her bed or chair. She ripped the window shades and used the curtain tiebacks as belts or neckties. Charlotte's being was a parallel of the condition of her own room. Her bedroom now looked more like a stripped down hotel room rather than the beautifully decorated bedroom it once was.

This thing called "Alzheimer's" just relentlessly keeps taking away one layer after another from the sufferer's persona and from what there is in life that they can appreciate and enjoy. Who would be left when there were no more layers to remove? How much more was there of Charlotte and how much more could we do for her?

It amazed me that when someone as attractive as Charlotte could become so angry, agitated and aggressive that I would look at her and actually see her as ugly. She was and still is a very, very beautiful woman, and how her entire face could take on the look of a wicked witch with her once playful, sparkling eyes narrowed and squinted with such disgust and mistrust startled me every time. What transforming power this disease has on everyone!

Alzheimer's takes the golden threads of who you are and tangles them into a knotted mass that cannot be untangled. This jumbled chaos, this person under the total siege of the disease, cannot be discounted and put aside. What about her golden threads? What about her spirit and her soul? What about what lies beneath her outer façade?

Often I looked at my favorite photo of Charlotte and only wanted to have her be as she was when that picture was taken. The photo was of Charlotte with an insert of Ray's baby picture. The photo was a gift from Charlotte to Ray's dad. It is so lovely and heartwarming; I treasure it. Charlotte was a beautiful, healthy young woman so full of life. This young woman, Charlotte, definitely could have been a "pin up girl" in some wartime service guy's heart. In fact, she was just that to Ray's dad when he was overseas in World War II. In my eyes, she was a 1940s version of Bernadette Peters. Is it not so that we often reminisce of how things used to be and long for those times once again?

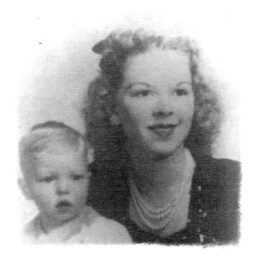

*"Charlotte with Ray in 1944"*

Why did it have to come to be so cruelly different now?

At times, for me, Charlotte's outward appearance and behaviors overpowered any glimpse of her golden threads. It seemed, at times, that I was like the jailor who had to keep Charlotte under some kind of control. Those circumstances made it more difficult for me to maintain a tender relationship with her. Our Matthew, Kelsey, Kayla, and even Marley were more able to interact with Charlotte's spirit and ignore the other stuff. So many times each of them touched Charlotte in that deep place where the real person remained.

Kelsey would share her coloring books with Charlotte. She would sit and color with Great-Grandmom and encourage her to use more colors and talk to her about the pictures. Charlotte did not seem to be able to understand most of the words that Kelsey spoke to her, but Charlotte certainly did feel the precious gift of being accepted with no judgments or criticism.

Kelsey would ask her simply what color the apple was or what color the sun was as she pointed to them. Charlotte would guess red or yellow or whatever color she thought it was, sometimes getting it correct, then Kelsey's face would light up and the hoorays would abound. Great-Grandmom got it right! Charlotte's joy was obvious through her laughter.

If Charlotte was still coloring when Kels was finished, she would not leave Great-

Grandmom there by herself; she'd just get her book and read until Charlotte was finished coloring. The two of them coloring and reading at our kitchen table became a beautiful study in one generation growing in her knowledge and one generation losing her knowledge.

Our Kayla would pull up a chair beside Charlotte's chair. She would sit as close as she could to Great-Grandmom. Kayla's soft, sweet, tiny hand rubbing Charlotte's cheek will be a memory that I pray I never lose. Kayla and Charlotte's eyes would meet and the most luminous glow appeared on both of their faces. Smiles reinforced the moment, especially as Charlotte would tilt her head toward Kayla's face and rest it there so peacefully.

For me this was a sacred moment when Charlotte's golden threads were being tied in poofy, joyful bows. What a gift these children are to Charlotte! What a gift children are to all of us.

I might backtrack a bit and tell you that Ray's mom was not a "doting grandmother" to our sons. I guess that is why I am so deeply touched by what has happened with Matthew and Charlotte's relationship since Alzheimer's has set in.

There were times when my upbeat veneer did slip, especially in Matthew's presence. I would quickly mention some behavior that was driving me crazy, and Matthew would so gently remind me that Grandmom could not help herself. After the initial insult-to-injury pout, I was grateful for his calm reminder. I needed that tug back into the reality of the situation to be removed from the "poor me" place I wanted to go.

Matthew would sit and kid with her. He was able to make her laugh, and she felt comforted by his presence. From the very beginning of her decline, when we told Charlotte that we were going out for the evening, she would ask in such a needy voice, "Is Matthew going to be here?" As soon as we said that he would be, she was calm and content. I am proud of how tender Matthew is toward his grandmother. He remembers the good times they have had in the past, even though they may not have been as many as I would have wanted for them. It is the remembered love that sustains this part of their relationship and what a gift it is for both of them.

A big change that greatly affected us was when Charlotte, who loved being by herself, no longer wanted to be alone anytime. Her paranoid behavior became full fledged, so we had Charlotte in our presence whenever she was awake. It came on slowly, but my feelings of resentment came on very quickly. I wrestled with this resentment. When it came over me, I would fight so hard. I did not want to own this resentment. Covering it up with a smile and upbeat attitude became difficult at times. More of my freedom, more of our life was slipping away from me—from us.

"Lord, let me do this cheerfully," I would pray. This inner battle between wanting to be a cheerful giver and the resentment building up over having my life, my privacy and my home literally kidnapped created a persona like a topsy-turvy doll with a happy face on one side and the crying face on the other. I might have a negative feeling, but I kept it covered and would flip myself over and only show others my forced smile and "I can handle this" attitude.

Charlotte's transition into needing to be in our company all of the time was, for me, the most difficult development with which I had yet to cope. I was smothered by Charlotte's presence; at times I did not think that I could breathe.

It was hard on all of us in the evenings. Ray and I both liked to watch the news, but this was not good for Charlotte—many reports upset her—she could not distinguish that what she saw on the television was not happening to her. Ray's job was to use the remote and find the animal shows or some cartoon shows. Ray often said that if he had to watch one more "most amazing animals" show, he would scream or start growling!

Charlotte would sit in her chair if we were in her sight. We always made it possible for her to see us. If she lost sight of us, she would start to take off. We were like guard dogs keeping her in the designated area.

Charlotte was on a plateau in her Alzheimer's descent. Her behaviors had remained somewhat constant for quite a while and we were becoming better equipped to handle her. I was using many techniques I used in my classroom when I was teaching Kindergarten to deal with Charlotte. I knew that being proactive got better results than just being reactive.

I had such good support from the adult day care center. Many mornings after dropping Charlotte off, I sought out the nurses, social workers and caregiver staff to let them know what was going on with Charlotte. They always offered me a listening ear and helped me to feel confident in how I was handling things.

In fact, they even asked if I would write down some of the "little every day techniques" I used with Charlotte. They were always willing to use my techniques with her while she was at the center.

Routines at home had become a way of life now, and from my point of view, things were okay. I did not add up the minutes or the hours that were dedicated to Charlotte's well being. I was coping—I was able to put one foot in front of the other and get by each day.

I was fortunate not to have to work outside the home. My schedule was flexible and able to accommodate all of Charlotte's needs. This manageable state of affairs allowed our life to go on. Ray went to work every day and even played an occasional game of golf.

I belonged to a garden club, and I went to a yoga class on Monday mornings after I dropped Charlotte off at the center. Ray and I were still able to be active in our church ministry. Each of these activities in their own way fed me emotionally, physically and spiritually. I know, without a doubt, that unless you are fed, you cannot feed others.

# ♥ Chapter Ten...

## Medications

*"I found that keeping a notebook with the daily meds given, along with a written description of Charlotte's behavior in the morning, afternoon, evening and nighttime was extremely important."*

I needed to constantly be on guard, keep track of meds (what worked and what did not), juggle schedules, lose sleep, make arrangements for caregivers other than when Charlotte was at the center, keep up with the "clean sweeps" of her room and still carry on with our lives. Ray had taken over most of the food shopping and all of the financial and household matters because my time was filled taking care of Charlotte's needs. Because we both had some outside activities, we did not realize what our life at home had become. I was oblivious to what I actually considered "a normal life" at home. Ray had a much clearer picture of the reality of the state of our home life.

This is what I had come to know as "normal." I wanted Ray to get his sleep at night as he had to get up at 5:30 a.m. each morning. Ray has a very demanding job and he needs a clear and alert mind to manage all the duties for which he is responsible. We usually got Charlotte settled by 11:00 p.m. and then fell into bed, so that when Ray's head hit the pillow, he usually was dead to the world until the alarm went off. Charlotte woke up several times each night, and I would go and tend to her while Ray slept.

I took Charlotte for her routine check-up and talked with the doctor about her not sleeping. He wrote out a prescription for sleeping pills. Oh, I was so hopeful for a good night's sleep. That night after getting Charlotte settled down, I quietly left her room. It reminded me of when our boys were little, and we had to tiptoe out of their rooms at night. I locked the gate and fell into bed. I was really tired after not having much sleep many nights before. I do not even think that there was time for me to get my pillow in the desired position when a loud thud came from Charlotte's room. I jumped from our bed and in two giant steps was at the gate and unlocked it in a split second. There I found a drowsy, unhurt Charlotte on the floor; she had just rolled off the bed.

I managed to get her back into bed, placing pillows on the edge of the bed to help keep her from falling out. Except for locking the gate, the same routine of my getting back into bed was repeated. I knew from past experience that sleep would not be mine tonight; the probability of getting up and checking would be the night's agenda.

Sure enough, a while later, another thump, another leap, another sprint with the same end result. Charlotte was again on the floor. It seemed that the medicine was working; it was calming her down. But now she was so relaxed that whatever it is that keeps all of us from rolling out of bed at night was gone from Charlotte.

The rest of that night was spent with me sitting in a chair by the side of her bed. It reminded me of one of my mother's favorite songs with the lines, "Side by side, through all kinds of weather." Here we were, Charlotte and I, side by side. (The sleeping pills worked that night but then the very next night they had no effect at all.) This is the way it seemed to go with the several types of sleeping pills that were prescribed. Interrupted-sleep nights like this were the "norm."

Charlotte was now assessed as being in the very middle or moderate stages of the disease. This is where *the "executive function"—the ability to initiate, sustain, and stop activities and to be mentality flexible really become non-existent.*[1-3] Charlotte was mentally inflexible a good part of the time. She was becoming unable to adapt to the circumstances around her. She could be very rigid and it was difficult to get her to comply with what she needed to do. Obstinate would be a good word to describe her behavior for the most part. No one could tell us how long this stage would last. The biggest concern that I had was how to keep Charlotte manageable so she could attend the adult day care center every day.

Reports from the center were that her behavior was becoming more aggressive and agitations were becoming more pronounced, more frequent. I got the report in the morning when I dropped Charlotte off at the center, and Ray got the scoop when he picked her up in the afternoon after work.

After taking Charlotte to her doctor, she was put on Lorazapam[2] in small doses to help curb her agitation and aggression.

Another new medicine, Namenda,[3] was also prescribed. Unlike some of the other medicines that had been tried in the past and which only worked once and then made no improvement, these new meds did help.

When Charlotte was uncooperative about taking her meds, the trick of putting her medicine into applesauce or ice cream was used. I also found a way to give her those small Lorazapam[2] pills when she was obstinate and resistant to taking them. I wet the pill, and stuck it to one side of a lollipop and then offered it to her with the other side showing toward her. That really worked great.

I did have to experiment with the Lorazapam[2] a bit, as I did not want Charlotte groggy but did want her calmer. There is a fine line getting just the right dose. It takes time and patience to keep track of what impact the medicine has on the person taking it and then getting back with the doctor to keep him informed. Working with a doctor this closely can really do so much to find the best distribution and dosage of medicine for the patient.

Keeping a notebook with the daily meds given, along with a written description of Charlotte's behavior in the morning, afternoon, evening and nighttime was extremely important. When speaking with the doctor, I did not have to try to rack my brain about what I thought occurred. It was so good to have this type of written log in front of me. Keeping this kind of record, gave me confidence and a sense of being able to stay on top of things.

| Date: / / | | |
|---|---|---|
| Medicine: | Comments | Questions for doctor |
| Morning: | | |
| Noontime: | | |
| Dinnertime: | | |
| Bedtime: | | |

*"Keeping a record"*

Being able to give and receive good detailed information is one of the biggest assets in doing the very best that can be achieved for a loved one's care. Even though I may fear that I sound "dumb" because I keep asking the same question over and over,

I MUST understand the doctor's answer. If I do not get it, then the doctor will have to explain it again until I do get it.

It is also true for the doctors, so I know that they understand me. They must be clear on the information that I am relaying to them. This is truly the greatest challenge for anyone advocating for a patient's good health care. It is hard for me to ask the doctor to, please, repeat what he or she thought I was saying about a particular issue. When I get their interpretation then I know if we are on the same page with communication. Some of the doctors look at me as if I have four eyes and no ears, but I know how imperative it is for them to understand exactly what I am saying to them.

When taking Charlotte into the center each morning, I usually had an upbeat attitude because we were documenting her progress, or perhaps it would be more accurate to say regression, together. I saw that this method of record keeping had played a part in getting her settled down and was hoping that the center was also seeing the progress that she was experiencing.

I have to admit, though, that each time I went in the front door of the center, I held my breath. What kind of report would they give to me? Charlotte had been asked to leave two other centers, and I always had that in the back of my mind. Would she be told that she could not attend this center anymore as well? Then what would we do?

# ❤ Chapter Eleven...

## Sleep Issues

*"The first really 'out of control' bedtime episode with Charlotte resulted in a 911 call for help, as we just could not physically handle her."*

*Spring and early summer 2004*

Charlotte had an appointment to go to a new Alzheimer's facility for an evaluation. It was an affiliate of Johns Hopkins Hospital. The appointment was about 10 weeks away. I wanted to make sure that everything that was known to be of help to the Alzheimer patient was available for Charlotte. All that we had to do was to wait. Waiting is not an easy thing to do with someone in Charlotte's fragile state. She was so up and down, with some things working for her and others failing miserably.

In June, 2004, celebrating another high school reunion, my classmate was telling us about their next cruise, which would be to Alaska in August.

Ray had always wanted to make this trip. August 1 would be our 40$^{th}$ anniversary, and we had not made any special plans. What a wonderful present this would be for Ray and me—a cruise to Alaska!

We wanted to do this, and I worked hard to make the respite plans for Charlotte and to finalize our travel arrangements. This was no small task because of the short time span between that night of the reunion in June and the departure day for Alaska.

Reservations for respite were somewhat limited and filled up quickly, especially in the summer months. We were only able to find split time-slots at two facilities. This plan also involved my sister Jean's generosity in transporting Charlotte to and from one respite place to the adult day care center each day.

All of the plans were finalized by the end of June. Although I was concerned about not being able to find one place for Charlotte to stay the entire time we would be gone, it was all arranged. We were going to have a dream come true—a 40$^{th}$ anniversary cruise.

The new meds Charlotte had been given were working better during the day. Everything was falling into a "normal" routine once again. But it was only a couple of weeks until another problem raised its ugly head.

The already testy bedtime situation became an even bigger problem. Charlotte's paranoia and aggression increased greatly, and she would get herself so wound up that it would take hours to settle her down with no real change until the medicine finally took hold or she just plain wore out.

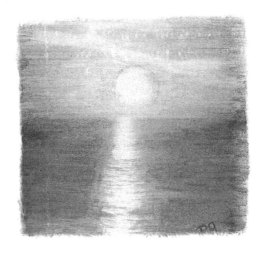

*" The sun going down is a beautiful sight, yet it can signal the beginning of a terrible night for the Alzheimer's patient. "*

The label that is put on this kind of behavior is called "sundowning." Some Alzheimer's patients demonstrate this kind of behavior after the sun goes down. All of their fears seem to magnify, and they become explosive and uncontrollable. This could definitely describe Charlotte's actions at this point at bedtime. If we tried to soothe her, she would jerk herself away from us and thrash about and strike out, as if she were going to hit us. The more we tried to talk to her, the worse she seemed to get.

A nurse practitioner stated that "sundowning" syndrome seems to heighten in November, when there is the shortest amount of daylight and continues until well after Christmas. Charlotte had been a sun worshipper and I still wonder if the lack of being out in the sun on a daily basis contributed to her having this syndrome.

Ray's presence in her room only seemed to exacerbate the situation. Charlotte would begin using vulgar expressions. Many of her ramblings contained language that I had not heard before, but her inflection and tone made me think of movie scenes in "The Exorcist."

The first really "out of control" bedtime episode with Charlotte resulted in a 911 call for help, as we just could not physically handle her. She kicked, screamed, swatted at us and truly scared us. After about two hours of this intense commotion with no sign of letting up, Ray called 911. Ray and I could not take another minute of this without some intervention. Both of us were drained and exhausted, hardly able to function. Charlotte was taken by ambulance, still ranting and raving, and was admitted to the hospital. She had to be put in restraints to be managed. It was a terrible night until she was given several different concoctions to calm her down. What this must have been like for her, I cannot imagine.

Charlotte was given many different tests, including a CAT scan. It showed no strokes, no other reason to explain this kind of uncontrollable behavior. The tests also showed that Charlotte did not have a UTI infection this time.

It was several hours until Charlotte calmed down; the vest type restraint was still being used to keep her in bed. She was much calmer. The loud, violent, aggressive behavior was no longer present. She did keep up her mutterings but was so much better on the whole. When Charlotte was being released two days later, Ray asked the nurse if he could take the restraint vest home. She said that was fine. It had worked so well to keep her in bed and she did not seem to be bothered by it. It would be a good thing to have on hand so that she would not fall out of bed and hurt herself.

When we got Charlotte home, all of the hospital things like the plastic tub, opened tubes of cream, and such were put under the bathroom sink, including the vest.

Charlotte had a couple of rather uneventful days, and with her music, bedtime was working out pretty well. She got up a few times, but was easily put back into bed. We took the bedrails off the bed that our granddaughter, Kayla used and put them on Charlotte's bed. They worked until a few nights later when Charlotte was out of bed once again. She had scooted out by the foot of the bed, bypassing the side rails. Oh, the hope of things being better was once again denied us. How much more could we take? Ray was so concerned that I was getting so little sleep. Sleep—sleep— a good night's sleep is what I prayed for.

I remembered the vest that the hospital had used to keep Charlotte in bed and decided to give it a try at home. It worked beautifully. It was a mesh vest that zippered in the back and had two long straps on each side of the waistband. The strap was tied to the bedrail loosely, as I wanted to make sure that Charlotte could turn over and sit up in bed, if she wanted. It did keep her from getting out at the bottom of the bed. I finally had some peace of mind.

Now when Charlotte woke up and called out, I would go in and tend to her. If she needed to use the bathroom, I was able to take her and not be concerned about her getting up by herself and being unsteady on her feet because of the effects of the meds. The music, the bedrails and the vest were good things.

Again, anything that I could come up with worked for a certain period of time. Then I had to go back to the drawing board for another idea. The regular bedtime scenario continued for about two weeks or so. I was in contact with the doctor, still trying to get some nighttime relief for both Charlotte and me but to no avail. Once again, the hope I had for a good night's sleep went out the window.

Charlotte had been very quiet this particular bedtime. Through the intercom, I could hear her moving around and even heard her body against the bedrail. I knew all of the sounds by heart but heard nothing that made me have to get up out of bed. After a bit Charlotte began her soft mutterings, and I just kept listening, praying that it would not get any more involved. It was not to be. All of a sudden, the intuition kicks in and you just know that things are not right. I got up and cautiously walked into Charlotte's room. I could not believe my eyes. It was the most harrowing night I had witnessed so far. Charlotte had removed all of her nightclothes from the waist down. She even pulled the diaper off and for lack of a better word "trashed" her bed and all around it with her feces. (She was continent during the day, but used a diaper at night.) This was my "rock bottom" and finally, finally, at that moment, I saw the enormity of the situation that we faced. That I faced!

After I had cleaned Charlotte and her room, she finally settled down around 3:00 a.m. I was so frustrated and borderline hysterical that I went down to the computer and wrote a note to her doctor. I wrote that note thinking that no one really understood what we were going through. I needed to be heard. I needed help. We needed help.

If only the doctor would prescribe the correct medicine, this could be resolved. I was worn out and sent a fax off to Charlotte's long-time doctor. Being at my wits end, this note could very well be labeled a "gripe" session. It detailed every action that had taken place with regard to Charlotte's behavior that night. I was venting. I pleaded for his help with this ongoing situation.

The kind doctor responded to the fax by calling Ray first and then calling me. He told me in no uncertain terms that I was not Nancy Reagan with a household staff and that I could not continue to take care of Charlotte on my own. She needed to be placed in an Alzheimer's unit. He also reamed me out for using the vest restraint on Charlotte. He told me restraints were not allowed to be used. He reiterated that Charlotte needed to be placed in an Alzheimer's facility.

Then the good doctor suggested that we were keeping Charlotte with us more for my own benefit than for hers. Ray had told him how committed I was to caring for Charlotte until the end. I fought off his suggestions. I paid no heed to his telling me what the best thing was for Charlotte. Why was I so determined to keep doing this on my own? My focus was on how in the world could Charlotte's being with strangers be better than being at home? No, relinquishing Charlotte to someone else's care, releasing ourselves from what I believed to be our duty, was not in my heart.

I truly believed that if she just got the right medicine, things would be okay. I believe that people, in general, are hopeful and hope-filled. I know I kept hoping that Charlotte could get better. Well, realistically not better from Alzheimer's, but better controlled so that we could handle her. It just did not sink in that there was no getting better for her. How complicated, debilitating and frightening Alzheimer's truly was just escaped my comprehension. I kept tilting at windmills.

In the light of day, I began trying to deal with the reality that I had finally faced the previous night. My body shook with the reality of what I had witnessed. What could I do to help Charlotte? Please, Lord, help her and help me.

The bedrails were kept; the restraining vest thrown away. I have since learned that some legal experts would label using the restraining vest as elder abuse—illegal imprisonment. There is so much of which the ordinary person is unaware.

It took a few days for me to recover from this last episode. In fact, I am still not fully recovered and maybe never will be. How could this happen? How does a person get so out of it? How can our bodies and minds treat "us" so badly?

It was getting harder and harder to wait for Charlotte's appointment at the new Alzheimer's facility. That was my new hope; that was the brass ring I needed to grab. As I put all of this down on paper, it was so clear to me how much I was in (to use a now politically incorrect phrase from my childhood) an "Indian Giver" mode. I gave in to the enormity of the situation at that moment and said, "I give up!" In just a short time, I would take that surrender right back. I began to look for another source of rescue that would help us to keep Charlotte in our home.

Immediately after this traumatic episode, another visit to websites dealing with Alzheimer's revealed the following shocker: "Caregivers want the AD patient given medication that knocks them out for twelve hours at night and a restraint to keep them in bed!" There I was on the screen! That is what I wanted, except I was only hoping for six or seven hours of sleep for Charlotte (and for me), not twelve, so was I so bad?

Pondering these words on the screen, another tiny sliver of awareness crept into my mind. Deep inside of me hope would not, could not, die. I would somehow be able to stick to my plan of taking care of Charlotte until the end. If I could just get over these losing battles, I might be able to win the war. How naïve! How bewildered and self-deceiving I was!

There is always something to be learned in everything that happens, and it just took us, and especially, me, a long, long time to learn from the lessons before me. One helpful lesson that I did learn was to use a jumpsuit garment on Charlotte at bedtime. It was a one-piece, zippered in the front, with leg holes that I put on backwards over her pajamas with the zipper in the back. This worked really well. She was unable to remove any of her clothes. It is worth mentioning here how important it was for us to use these "helpful hints" such as the jumpsuit when Charlotte was in her cooperative state, before the "sundowning" showed its agitated signs. I would rub the soft material of the jumpsuit on her face and talk about it being so "comfy" and she was receptive to putting it on.

The time that I spent with Charlotte as I prepared her for bed was usually good. I think that she loved having my undivided attention. We were the only ones upstairs and she did not have to compete for my focus. It was a good chunk of time that there were no interruptions from any one else, and somehow I believe that, on some level of comprehension, Charlotte realized that she had me all to herself. She liked that scenario.

# ♥ Chapter Twelve...

## Hope for the Hopeless

*"I needed shared 'tidbits of survival' skills, not only for the one suffering with the disease, but also for the family suffering with them."*

Summer 2004

Passing by the television, I heard that Oprah was having a show about Alzheimer's disease. My body locked into stillness, as if someone had yelled, "freeze!" My eyes peered at the screen, scanning for any written message; my ears strained and my frazzled, almost worn out, department of hope fluttered.

For the past four years, whether I desired it or not, my mind, body and soul seemed to be yanked and pulled into those two words—Alzheimer's Disease. I suspect that dealing with sickness of any kind on a day-to-day basis causes this kind of knee-jerk reaction to the slightest mention of the illness from which you or your loved one suffers.

Perhaps there are those who try to avoid any mention of illness with as much intensity. I am definitely the information seeking junkie type. Any program on TV or on the radio relating to Alzheimer's gets my full attention. I read books, newspapers and magazine articles with great interest and attention to detail.

I eagerly awaited the July 13, 2004 upcoming Oprah show. It was the one with Maria Schriver telling the story of her dad, Sargent Schriver, having Alzheimer's. Maria wrote the book, "What's Happening to Grandpa?" It is a beautifully written book that I have read to our granddaughters several times. The show also included Leeza Gibbons who shared her mother's battle against Alzheimer's disease. Both of these women use their resources to help raise money and educate others about the urgent need for research. I sat mesmerized by their stories, relating to much of what they shared.

At the end of the show, I was slumped over, wanting more—needing so much more. I was so hoping to hear how their families handled things on a day-to-day basis. I needed shared "tidbits of survival" skills, not only for the one suffering with the disease but also for the family suffering with them.

It came to me that possibly these celebrities' father and mother, respectively, were in the early stages of Alzheimer's and day-to-day survival was not such a desperate issue for them yet. It is also true that these families have many more resources than the average family. Tears filled my eyes, as another hope-filled expectation went unmet. I immediately went to the computer and sent an e-mail message to Oprah stating my thoughts and feelings about how much more I had hoped to get from the show.

Weeks later, on another Oprah show, I saw a woman who wrote in telling how another woman's story had kept her from taking her life when she was so depressed. Oprah invited her to come in person to share this and as she began to talk, her voice quivered as the tears fell from her eyes. Her desperation and pain came from caring for her mother, who has Alzheimer's. I trembled at each word she had the courage to get out. My heart ached so much for her. She did not go into any description of her troubles, but she did not have to speak a word about her daily struggle. I believed that I knew what she was trying to handle. What do ordinary people do to care for their loved one with Alzheimer's?

I continued to surf the web, read any book or articles I could find, and tried to find some survival techniques—all without much success. It was a real challenge to find detailed information, and I often thought of those with fewer resources who may neither have access to information nor the energy to search for it, especially the elderly spouse caring for his or her husband or wife. The spouse with Alzheimer's is the "squeaky wheel" who gets all of the attention while the other partner's needs are neglected, often leading to illness or even the death of the caregiver. What on earth do these caregivers do to get through each and every day?

Not needing another task, I nonetheless, felt compelled to try and share our day-to-day dealings with this disease. Being driven by the need for information and a stronger drive to share information, I decided after watching the Oprah show that I was going to try and share our story—our struggle—relating to Alzheimer's. I wanted to offer some helpful information on day-to-day living with Alzheimer's. I also thought that people on the outside could never comprehend the seemingly endless day-to-day, minute-to-minute struggle that the patients and caregivers go through each day. Even doctors and other professionals, unless directly affected by Alzheimer's personally, do not understand. Family members who are not involved in this day-to-day, totally immersing cycle cannot understand either. I decided that I would write a book sharing our struggles for and with Charlotte and would try to offer some sort of assistance to others going through the same thing with their loved one.

# ♥ Chapter Thirteen...

## A Transformation

*"Charlotte had no control of her own body and mind, and I did not have any control over Charlotte or this illness."*
*Summer 2004*

Despite all that I knew, had been told and was living through, I still went for a while longer doing the best that I could and believing that I could keep Charlotte in our home.

Charlotte's bedtime seemed like a never-ending battle that I needed to win if my goal for her care was to be achieved. One bedtime episode scared me so badly that I thought that there was the possibility that she might not be able to come out of the paranoia and aggression into which she fell, and then what would we do?

Ray and I were with Charlotte in her room, but nothing we tried to do worked to calm her. Ray called Matthew up to see if his presence would help as Ray always got the brunt of Charlotte's anger, and he did not want to antagonize this volatile situation in any way.

Ray paced in the hallway out of sight—not out of mind—as Matthew and I tried different things to calm Charlotte. Charlotte was letting out these primal screams from deep down inside of her. Her shrieks went right through me. The atmosphere was absolutely surreal. Her whole body just kept jerking, seizure-like, and her words were jumbled and discordant, making no sense at all. The words, the bits of words she could manage to say were spit out as if they had been chewed up. She flailed her arms and legs. We were invisible to her; she screamed right past us; she had no idea of where she was or who she was.

It took Matthew on one side of her and me on the other to keep her from getting out of bed. Bed was the safest place for her. This was such a hard, hard time for Charlotte to endure and for us to witness.

As the evening progressed, or rather regressed, I was hard-wired into panic mode. I could not stop having thoughts about our upcoming vacation. Everything was a go and now this latest episode could put a halt to everything. I judged that my focus should have been on Charlotte's needs, and yet it was thoughts of our Alaskan vacation that kept creeping into my mind. The guilt was starting to choke me.

Matthew was Charlotte's god-send that night (and Ray's and mine too). His voice was soothing as he just repeated over and over, "We're right here, Grandmom." He gently rubbed her arm and kept the soothing mantra of his words, softly spoken and calming.

Charlotte was so helpless and pitiful in this state. You could not help but be moved by the torture she was experiencing. My tears were so bittersweet that night—remorseful for what Charlotte was going through and at the same time, tears of gratitude for the wonderful caring man willing to go through this, with and for his grandmother. Tasting the salt of my own tears reminded me that Matthew is a salt-of-the-earth kind of person. What a compassionate man! How proud Ray and I are that Matthew has this beautiful quality.

The next morning a frantic call was made to the Hopkins' Alzheimer's facility to see if they could reschedule Charlotte's appointment any earlier for her evaluation. I told them how she was going downhill so quickly, and I was desperate for some help and asked for any earlier time slot they might have to see Charlotte.

It was bad news. They were completely booked and the woman on the other end of the phone added that she was getting so many calls for this same type of situation that she had nothing to offer. Charlotte could not be seen until her scheduled appointment and that was not for another two weeks. Waiting is so difficult when you need to be rescued.

However, in this most dreadful time, something truly amazing happened. It was when Charlotte was at her most vulnerable that she opened my heart unequivocally. I left the "respectful only" mode somewhere in the chaos of the agony she was suffering. My heart fully accepted this woman, my mother-in-law, Ray's mother, our sons' grandmother, our granddaughters' great-grandmother and most importantly, this child of God. I cannot fully describe what took place. It transcends my human understanding.

I can tell you that somewhere in all of that late night misery, the resentment, the duty and obligation I had felt before, and really did not want to openly acknowledge, diminished. It left me. It must have been consumed by the compassion and empathy that washed over me and filled in each one of my cracks of judgments and resentments.

After Charlotte's meds kicked in that night, and she was safely tucked into bed with a soft snoring purr emitting from her quieted lips, my tears resumed in greater abundance. As I looked on this now peaceful, sleeping body, my heart could only absorb the tragic life she now had to endure. These tears were reserved solely for this woman who was suffering so terribly.

I left Charlotte's room and locked the gate. Slowly, heavily, I walked our short hallway, which seemed a city-block long. I fell into the comfort of my own bed and cried quietly for this poor tormented soul. That was when my transformation took place. I get it! I got it! As Oprah says: an "ah ha moment!" As I look back, I believe this moment was the first time that I let go and let God in.

Charlotte is NOT responsible.

How very difficult it is to truly come to that realization—to believe it—even though it is obvious.

A dire tug of war waged inside of me. In my mind, I could visualize the kid's game played with a big rope. On one side was Charlotte's negative acting out and all of my "control" that I wanted over her behaviors and, on the other side, all of the knowledge that I had about Alzheimer's and its dreadful results. The tug of war ended; no more pulling or tugging. Both my mind and my heart were finally in sync. I could stop fighting it.

Nothing about this illness is Charlotte's fault. She had no control of her own body and mind, and I did not have any control over her or this illness. Alzheimer's might take Charlotte's mind and, eventually, her body, but never her soul. Her suffering, her unbelievably difficult existence living with Alzheimer's for so long is certainly more than enough to make up for any shortcomings I ever judged that she possessed. Charlotte is living a purgatory right now living with Alzheimer's.

I seemed to have been graced with some new inner strength and understanding that I had previously lacked. If only I could have received complete acceptance of the reality of Alzheimer's and the disastrous course it navigates on its victim and the people who love them and are close to them.

This beautiful awareness that was gifted to me did not make what was yet to come any easier to handle. In fact, I believe it made it all the more difficult for me. This gift came with intense emotional strings attached. Up until then, I knew that I had given Charlotte the same kind of physical care that I would have given to my own mother, had she been the Alzheimer's victim, but I was unable to release true compassion for Charlotte. It was my restrictive attitude, my holding onto long-held feelings of obligation versus empathy for her that had been changed in the transformation.

I had been devoted to my mom and adored her, but I did not have that same depth of feeling for Ray's mom. I can honestly say now that I do not believe that I could have had more compassion or empathy for my own mother than I have for Charlotte today.

I began to see this gut-wrenching cycle of torment that Charlotte was going through at this time and wondered if this was not her last desperate cry for rescue. Did Charlotte know that the disease was taking her over and was this her only way of fighting it? Was this her final effort to claw her way out of the jaws of Alzheimer's?

I believed that somewhere deep inside she had an awareness—some instinct—that she was losing the battle. Alzheimer's was taking her alive!

Somehow, all of us got through the next two weeks, which are all a blur to me, until our appointment at the new Alzheimer's facility. There Charlotte and I met with a great team of evaluators who concurred with all of the earlier assessments. Charlotte did indeed have Alzheimer's. She was moving from the middle into the latter stage. *A person in the third or latter stage of AD becomes so debilitated as to be especially vulnerable to infectious disease; most commonly, people with severe AD die of bronchitis or pneumonia (Beard, Kokman, Sigler et al. 1996; National Institute of Aging 2000, at 6).* [1-4]

*The ordinary course from AD onset to death has been estimated as a period of seven to ten years (Mace and Rabins 1999, at 291). A recent analysis of a Canadian population, however, observed that the median survival from the onset of AD "is much shorter than has previously been estimated," a bit more than three years (Wolfson, Wolfson, Asgherian et al. 2001). Nevertheless, "although some patients with [AD], particularly the oldest, may die within three years of receiving the diagnosis, many patients, particularly those in whom the onset occurs at an early age, live for a decade or more with the ravages of severe dementia" (Kawas and Brookmeyer 2001).* [1-5]

One thing that impressed me immensely was how the doctor listened to me. He had asked me to tell him about Charlotte and to describe a day with her. After I did that, the doctor said, "Okay, now this is what I heard you say." He then repeated back to me what I had just told him and waited for me to concur. Then he asked if her agitation during the day and her sleeping at night were my main areas of concern. Again, he waited for my reply. He really listened to me. In his office, I never felt rushed or hurried along—he had time to listen. So many doctors just do not seem to have the time to listen; they have such time restraints with being allotted only so many minutes per patient. This is how the system works and just how many gerontologists are there to handle the growing number of seniors?

The doctor gave the following information to us:

## 1. What is Dementia?

*In the past, terms like "senility," "organic brain syndrome" or "late life confusion" were used to describe the elderly person who had difficulty thinking and remembering. The understanding of what is normal aging and what is abnormal aging has progressed so that new terms are used.*

*The medical definition of dementia is the following:*

*A global decline in intellectual abilities of sufficient severity to interfere with occupational and or social functioning. This occurs in clear consciousness.*

*What does this mean?*

_Global decline_ means that more than one aspect of thinking is affected. So that a person who only has memory problems or who only has difficulty in speaking would not be described as demented. Persons who are demented often have difficulty in remembering, communicating, making decisions and planning.

_Sufficient severity_ to impair functioning means that the problems the patient has are severe enough to produce problems in their daily lives. Common problems include not remembering to pay bills, not being able to plan, shop and prepare meals, and getting lost in familiar places.

_Clear consciousness_ means that the person is awake and alert. This is in contrast to a person who is drowsy and not thinking properly due to an illness such as pneumonia and fever or who is impaired by medications, anesthesia or alcohol.

What causes dementia?

Some conditions can mimic dementia and must be identified and treated. These include depression, intoxication from medications both prescription and over the counter and herbs and thyroid disease among others.

*There are many causes of dementia. Some get worse over time and some do not. Causes include strokes, Parkinson disease, Huntington disease and many others. Alzheimer's disease is the most common cause. It can be diagnosed accurately and a variety of treatments are available.*

*2. Alzheimer's disease*

*Alzheimer's disease is the most common cause of dementia in later life. AD begins gradually and gets worse over a period of years. The common symptoms of AD begin with the letter A and are known as the 4 A's of AD. Each of the symptoms causes difficulty in daily life.*

*"Amnesia:" (Memory) AD causes difficulty in registering new memories and recalling them. Common examples include the patient asking the same question over and over and losing their belongings. These problems occur because the part of the brain involved in registering new memories is damaged.*

*"Aphasia:" (Language) AD impacts on the ability of the patient to communicate with others and to understand what is being said to them. Many patients develop difficulty in finding words and their speech becomes vague and empty. Second, patients will have difficulty in understanding what is being said to them. Language problems are frustrating for both the patient and caregiver.*

123

*"Apraxia:"* *(Doing things) AD damages the parts of the brain that are involved in planning and directing the body to do things. Common examples are putting on clothing backwards and picking up food with their hands instead of using a knife and fork. Tasks must be simplified for the patient who has this symptom. Often, starting a task such as putting food on a fork and handing it to the patient can get a task started.*

*"Agnosia:"* *(Recognizing the world) Though patients with AD can see the world, brain disease causes difficulty in recognizing what they see. Common examples of this are the person who stands in front of the refrigerator looking at the milk but unable to recognize it. Some patients who may be unable to recognize their caregiver become uncooperative or run away.* [1-5]

The doctor said that the language symptom (Aphasia) was Charlotte's greatest weakness. She was capable of carrying on a conversation by herself, speaking in complete paragraphs filled with cohesive sentences making sense. This happened many times daily as she carried out her one-sided dissertations.

You could not interrupt or question her as to what she was saying. For Charlotte, there was no understanding of any question you asked. When spoken to, it must have been as if she were hearing a foreign

124

language. How frustrating and frightening this must have been for her. Charlotte basically only understood very simple words and needed hand gestures to get a response of some kind from her.

The doctor at this facility prescribed an antipsychotic medicine, Seroquel,[4] in a very low dose to be used with her Lorazapam[2] and Namenda,[3] At the time, I did not clearly understand that antipsychotic drugs needed to build up in a person's system and then be evaluated as to whether or not they are doing the job. I just wanted an instant medicine that would help Charlotte. It was hard to wait.

I stayed in close contact with the doctor through e-mail and phone calls every couple of days to fill him in on how Charlotte was doing. Her nighttime turmoil continued with a better night here and there. Overall, much more improvement was still desperately needed.

I was sleep deprived and the stress of caretaking was beginning to take a real toll on my body. For well over two years, a good night's sleep came only when Charlotte was in respite care.

For the last three months or more, most nights consisted of maybe two or three hours of restless sleep. Every night the intercom lay beside my pillow with the constant sounds from Charlotte's bedroom. Sleep never reached the deep restful body refueling level that every healthy mind and body need.

It was becoming more difficult for me to stay upbeat and cheerful, even though my attitude had been transformed. My body was screaming from the inside that something had to change; this could not keep going as it was. I was losing weight (not such a bad thing, I told myself), as I always seemed to be grabbing a quick bite from my dinner plate.

Charlotte ate earlier than our dinnertime, so if she would stir and start to get up out of her chair, off I would go. My eating could wait, but Charlotte could not.

After she was upstairs for the night, I would start running the steps. It would not be an exaggeration to say that I climbed them twenty times a night to attend to Charlotte (such good exercise, right?).

Our family time in the evenings sort of died. Matthew, Ray and I liked to play cards, Scrabble or other games, and those times were either constantly interrupted or squelched altogether. Ray was the one most able to admit his displeasure about all of this. He was the most open and honest about how much time it took from us, and especially me, to care for his mom.

Ray shared many times how grateful he was for how well I took care of Charlotte and told me how much he worried that it might be getting too much for me. I only wanted to hear his words of gratitude, not the words telling me about his worry. My mind was set. Our family, Ray, JR, Matthew and I, had cared for Daddy until he died. Ray and I took care of my sister, Be, until she died. I believed that we must give Ray's mother this same kind of care until her passing. I would accept nothing less. My letting go and letting God in was slipping away from me again.

# ♥ *Chapter Fourteen...*

### The Decision

*"I began to entertain the idea of Charlotte
going into assisted-living.
No, I would not! No, I could not!
A dire tug of war waged inside of me."*
*July 2004*

My concern about Charlotte's respite
care while we were to be gone for our eagerly
awaited cruise to Alaska was still a constant
weight on my mind and my heart. With
Charlotte being on these new meds and with
her terrible nighttime episodes, I was worried
that all of the shuffling around for her respite
care might be too much for her.

Charlotte was to stay with Yolanda,
who cared for Charlotte as I did. My sister,
Jean, would transport her each day to and
from this assisted-living house to the day care
center. If anything happened to Charlotte

while my sister was transporting her, Jean would be beside herself. How could I put this kind of responsibility on my sister?

I scurried around and found a large Alzheimer's facility that would be able to take Ray's mom for part of the time. It was a brand new place, and Ray went to see it and was impressed with the people with whom he spoke. The bonus was that they would transport Charlotte to her regular adult day care center everyday. There were some drawbacks. It was new to us and no one was familiar with Charlotte nor she with them. We would be gone for three weeks, and this was a long time. We had never before left Charlotte for that long.

There also was a conflict in the method or philosophy of this facility. While speaking with one of the staff about Charlotte's sleeping situation, they mentioned that most times they decrease the meds of their residents after they are there awhile. She continued, "If the residents want to stay up all night that is okay, because they have business to take care of." This was nothing I had heard before; everyone needs a restful night's sleep, don't they? I was unsure of Charlotte going to this place. Of course, her declining behavior was the biggest drawback for all of these changes. It was a good thing we had purchased travel insurance!

The words of Charlotte's longtime doctor's kept creeping into my head, "It would be better for Charlotte to be in an Alzheimer's facility." In addition, thoughts of Ray's concern for me and the toll that taking care of Charlotte was having on me had expanded to some of our family members and close friends. Should I now give some credence to their concerns?

From the time I knew Ray's mom, she always said that she would never live past forty. She was a cancer survivor. She had to have a hysterectomy right after Ray was born and had thyroid cancer after that, so she did have some real basis for her prediction. I would make a joke and flip a quip back to her that she would probably out-live me!

Suddenly this long-time banter between us became a true irony. Would my long-ago prediction be the correct one? Charlotte was physically very healthy. She was very mobile in spite of her arthritic knees and shoulders. She indeed could out live me. How much longer could I physically keep up this pace?

I began to entertain the idea of Charlotte going into assisted-living. No, I would not! No, I could not! A dire tug of war waged inside, tearing at me. I really did not want to bring it up with Ray. He had already spoken loud and clear that he was ready. Ray was more concerned for my well-being than I was. He did not have the determination that I had to stick with this until it was over. My personality is driven with the curse of perfectionism. My giving up as Charlotte's primary care giver would be out of the accepted rigid guidelines of perfection. Could I handle that? Could I live with that?

I pleaded, "Lord, please send a clear answer to this critical situation." This prayer was ever on my lips; however, it appears that I needed a "hit you on the head with a two-by-four" answer to get my attention, even though the answer was loud and clear to everyone around me.

I had another dimension to my dilemma. If we were indeed considering placing Charlotte in an assisted-living facility permanently, how could we put her in respite care for three weeks and then move her to another new facility.

This definitely was not a good idea. This could not be good for Charlotte. Too much change is hard on anyone, let alone someone in Charlotte's state.

Charlotte continued with her nighttime terror, with a better night here and there; still each day became a little harder to get through.

Recalling the incident of the past where I had "saved" Charlotte's life, I put myself in her present condition, knowing what her life had become, and I had to force some terrible thoughts from being finished in my mind. I am deeply committed to all life being sacred, however, here on this written page, I can ask—"Would it have been better if I had not been able to save Charlotte's life back then before she got to this stage of the disease?"

While Charlotte was at the center during the day, I would try to do all of the necessary household chores and keep up with the rest of our life, as well. My yoga class was my time for total relaxation and meditation. I fought anything that tried to interfere with the priority I needed it to be.

My life was so full of doing, that if I stopped for a minute to sit down, I fell asleep. It was my adrenaline that kept me going once Charlotte was home from the center.

On weekends, I was fueled with the added boost of energy that I get in times of need. This allowed me to still be a doer and disguise the exhaustion I was denying to those around me. "I am doing fine," was the answer for everyone who wanted to know.

The usual evening routine was that the intercom moved from my bedside to the table in our family room. With some music playing in her room, Charlotte could be quiet for a while when she first got into bed. I was always on guard listening for any sounds warning that she was trying to get out of bed.

When we had friends over, I was on edge as to when she might start spitting out vulgarities. It was not that our friends would not understand our situation, but it was embarrassing because I knew that I had to respond to Charlotte's outbursts, thus leaving our guests on their own.

Our summer routine included our caring for Kelsey and Kayla on Wednesdays and Thursdays. In summers past, often on Wednesday, one of the girls would ask if there could be a "sleep over." They would spend the night if it was all right with their mom and dad as it was always fine with Ray and me. We love our time with them, and sleepovers are so much fun.

When Kelsey said, "Grammy, can we have a sleepover tonight?" this particular Wednesday, I actually slumped down and pretended not to hear her. How could Kelsey, now age 8 and Kayla, age 7 spend the night and see and hear their great-grandmother rant, rave, curse, scream, kick and flail? Kelsey and Kayla were very accepting and understanding of Charlotte's little escapades during the day. I could usually distract them from most of her inappropriate behavior. But there was no way we could camouflage or explain to them Charlotte's bedtime behavior. It would scare Kelsey and Kayla and confuse them. I, in no way, wanted them exposed to that part of Charlotte. My heart was breaking as I kept avoiding the sleepover question.

Ray and I were very willing to give up our time for Charlotte, but now it seemed that we were going to have to give up entertaining our friends and having sleepovers with our darling granddaughters, too!

Ray and I talked often about the time we have to spend with our Kelsey and Kayla being so precious to us. Their wanting to "hang out" with us would not last forever. They were growing much too fast. Our time with them was passing much too quickly. We wanted to enjoy them as much as we could; this time in our lives could never be relived. Now, we were being forced to choose.

Adding it all up, I knew it was time. My heart was forced into going along with the decision to find a permanent residence for Charlotte because we did not want to put her in a three-week respite situation and then place her in an assisted-living facility permanently.

We had to move quickly. Again, I prayed, "Lord, please send a clear answer to this situation." I saw that God answered that prayer in more ways than one. It was clear that the time was now. The fact that I was forced to move quickly was the other answer. If not pushed into making a decision because of our trip to Alaska, God knows I would have dragged it out and prolonged the inevitable. I thank God for this set of circumstances, which was the catalyst to my being clearly aware of what had to be done.

Our first choice for Charlotte would have been where she had gone often for respite or to be a live-in resident at the adult day care center she attended. These are both top-notch facilities with very wonderful caregivers. Charlotte would be so well cared for at either of these places. We knew that neither of these places were an option for Charlotte. Neither one of these fine places could handle Charlotte with the level of nighttime care that she required nor her unpredictable daytime behavior.

I knew that I wanted Charlotte to be in a smaller facility, but in the interviews, when I spoke of Charlotte's sleep issues, they were very hesitant to take her. Some were very direct; some were just very vague in their answer to our request for placement. For the most part, none had a "night time staff" to handle someone in Charlotte's volatile state.

I went to see some larger facilities and knew right away that Charlotte would not do well in them. She would have too much free space to roam and get into trouble taking other people's things and who knows what else if she were not under constant observation.

One of the large facilities assured me that Charlotte would fit right in and made light of my concerns with reassurances. It was not until I asked to speak with the head nurse who would be in charge of Charlotte's care that the picture was made clear. When the nurse joined the administrative and marketing people, and I again described Charlotte's behavior, this time I was heard and understood. The nurse said that they were neither staffed nor set up to handle Charlotte at this stage of Alzheimer's. The administrative and marketing staff wanted to fill a vacant slot, but the actual caregivers were the only ones who truly knew what it was to take care of middle-to-advanced stage Alzheimer's patients.

On one thing, I was very clear. I was very upfront and honest about all of Charlotte's behaviors. I did not want Charlotte to be placed somewhere and then be told that she was not fitting in and would have to leave. Charlotte had gone through that with the senior centers, and I did not want her going through that with assisted-living places, too. This move from our home was going to be hard enough on all of us without having to do it more than once.

Several of the assisted-living facilities were familiar because of my previous legwork when looking into respite care for Charlotte. I visited five different facilities, and it came down to a little larger facility than planned, but they had a nighttime staff and that was important for Charlotte. I still had my concerns about there being a bit more roaming room, but I was assured by the staff that it would be fine, and I believed it was workable.

God kept answering my prayers, even when I forgot that I should continue asking. As I was making some of the final arrangements over the telephone with this new facility, a staff member put me on hold. When she came back on the line, I picked up some hesitancy in her questions. She would have to check some things out and get back to me. I was in disbelief with this "I'll get back to you." My mind raced and for some unknown reason, I placed one more call to a home I had visited some time back inquiring about respite care. When I spoke with the owner, I once again gave a description of Charlotte's behaviors in full and loving detail. The owner listened and stated that they had residents with many of the same issues. She did not give any indication that they would give up on Charlotte's sleep-time issues easily. When I told her that Charlotte was in the care of doctors at the Hopkins' AD facility, she was elated, as they work closely with that facility. They were already working with a nurse practitioner who came to their place every month to monitor their residents.

The owner also seemed confident that Charlotte's sleep issues would settle down in time, by continuing to work closely with The Johns Hopkins affiliate Alzheimer's program. That was the pearl of wisdom that swayed me to this assisted-living house. I went to see the facility once again to meet the owner and caregivers. It was not our home, but it was clean, tidy and seemed to fit Charlotte's needs for a small intimate setting where she would be supervised all the time.

There was a lovely sunroom looking out on a treed yard with a horse farm right behind it. Charlotte would love this kind of setting. Ray and I went back in the evening, and it was settled. Charlotte would go to this assisted-living facility.

In order to do the very best for Charlotte, it was decided that the sooner we could get her moved in, the better. This way we could be around for her adjustment time before we took off for our trip. There was so much paperwork: evaluations, TB test, doctors' reports, medicine/medical forms, financial and legal forms to be filled out. The owner of this home was so helpful, as was Charlotte's doctor and his staff and the Department on Aging, as well as the staff at Charlotte's future residence. It was as if the whole process was placed on a flying carpet. Everything landed at the right destination.

# ♥ Chapter Fifteen...

## A New Home for Charlotte

*"Ray found the courage to take his mother
to her new residence that afternoon.
It was done. Charlotte was there."*

*August 2004*

Three days later, Charlotte would be in her new home. Oh boy, that was and still is difficult for me to say—her new home. Charlotte's moving day was to be on Thursday.

Kelsey and Kayla helped me get many things together for Great-Grandmom on Wednesday. They were such a great help to me. We were in Charlotte's room packing her things in the suitcase and all the while silent tears kept falling from my eyes. The girls were so tender and caring with me. They would move close to me and rub my arm.

They never once told me that everything would be all right. That is a sentiment adults speak so easily. Children intuitively know that sometimes things will not be all right or do not have to be all right and that is just the way it is. This part of Charlotte's journey that I shared with her will never be all right. It may be what must be done because we could not keep up the around the clock care schedule that Charlotte required at this point.

Having our granddaughters with me forced me to keep my emotions somewhat under control. They helped me to keep it together, as I was resisting this change so strongly. After the suitcases were filled, we packed the car. Then Kelsey and Kayla decided that they would draw pictures for Great-Grandmom's new room. For me, the tears flowed constantly. I kept praying, "Lord, please help us to get through this."

After JR picked the girls up that afternoon, Ray and I had more tasks to accomplish such as picking up some of the forms and taking Charlotte for a new TB test and other last-minute requirements. The jammed schedule of the late afternoon and evening occupied my mind and kept my hurting psyche at bay.

Wouldn't you know it? That evening Charlotte went off to bed rather smoothly. She woke up a few times but was easily coaxed to stay in bed and go back to sleep. I could not sleep. The path from our bed to her bed was well used that night. I sat in Charlotte's chair in the dark room and listened to her familiar snore. I had no coherent thoughts. Everything seemed mixed up. There were so many feelings inside of me. It was as if I was flopping like a cement mixer, turning the sand, stones and water with each feeling possessing its own weight. The noise of the stones hitting the metal container was like the pounding thumps in my heartbeat. Slowly the thuds subsided; it was coming together. But it was not relief that I felt, it was the cement, such a heavy mass, weighing me down. I did not know if I could lift myself from her chair.

It was done.

The decision was made.

Tomorrow was the day that Charlotte would leave our home. I felt like such a failure—unable to keep her home with us. I do not want to be a quitter. At home or in my classroom, the words "I can't do it" would never be accepted without a "good attempt" first. I knew first hand that usually a good attempt at something meant dealing with initial failure, but in the end, if I tried hard enough, reasonably good results could be achieved. Now, I was quitting, giving up, saying, "I can't do it anymore!" But oh, how I tried. I really did try to keep Charlotte until her end.

Sitting there, I thought of the conversations with our JR and Matthew just days before when I asked for their thoughts and feelings about our placing their grandmother in assisted-living. They both said they understood and supported our decision. But we spoke of a "what if" and now it was a reality. Would they still be okay with it? Knowing that Charlotte would not sleep in her room again nor live with our family anymore, I sat in the darkness and cried.

The busyness of the morning ritual of getting Charlotte up, dressed, fed and to the center filled Thursday's early hours. JR, Kelsey and Kayla met me at the center when I took Charlotte there in the morning. The girls loved walking Charlotte into the center, which they did most Wednesdays and Thursdays. They eagerly guided her to her place at the table and put on her apron.

JR hugged and kissed us; then he went off to work. As I watched him leave, the tenderness he had always shown his grandmother flashed before me. His and Karen's life was full and busy, and they were not around as much as the rest of us, but JR never missed the opportunity to give Charlotte a hug and kiss and have some bit of teasing for her to enjoy. Charlotte was blessed by this grandson's gentleness.

Kelsey and Kayla stayed by Charlotte's side while I sought out the staff members, who were such a vital part of my support. I told them what we had done. They held me as I cried. They said all the right things about how much we had done for Charlotte, but deep within, it still was not all right!

The girls and I left the center and went back home to finish getting Charlotte's things packed and over to her new residence.

Kayla somehow did not completely realize that Great-Grandmom was going to stay at this new place permanently. It was not until I mentioned that Grampy and Uncle Matthew would take Great-Grandmom's recliner chair over to the new place later that evening that Kayla's big, round eyes widened and now tears were falling from those precious baby blues. Kelsey went over to comfort Kayla. Thank you, Kelsey for doing what I could not do. From then on, there was a non-stop flow of tears over which I had no control.

Ray and I had already decided that I would get his mom's things over to the new place before Charlotte arrived later in the afternoon. The car was filled with Charlotte's things and when Kelsey, Kayla and I pulled into the driveway of the soon-to-be permanent residence for Charlotte, I began to tremble. If it were not for the blessing of having my sweet, sweet girls with me, I may not have stepped out of the car. They were so patient with me.

Finally, the three of us were out of the car and knocked on the door of Charlotte's new residence. It was opened by the same woman that Ray and I had met before. She welcomed us in a very cordial manner. I managed to introduced Kelsey and Kayla to her. She then showed us to the room that was to be Charlotte's.

In the state that I was in, each dreaded step forward just got me farther into what I was now seeing as a cold and grayish dwelling. It was as if I was in one of those dark dungeons in a Grimm's fairytale. The people there were like the stern and stoic characters the Grimm brothers introduced to their readers. As we put Charlotte's things away in the small facility-provided dresser, and I looked around at her new surroundings, I remember thinking that maybe it was like this in Harry Potter's under-the-stairs-bedroom—dark and dingy. "Would I want to live here?" were words that flashed like strobe lights in my head. I knew that answer for sure. No way! Of course not! (I was making that assessment from my present state of being—healthy, both in mind and body—or relatively so!)

My fear-filled imagination was so out there, so off-the-wall, that I truly know that if it had not been that Kelsey and Kayla were with me, I just might have bolted. It seems surreal as I look back on that afternoon. I did not even feel my tears anymore. I placed Charlotte's favorite quilt on her bed along with her pillow. The girls placed their precious drawings on her bed.

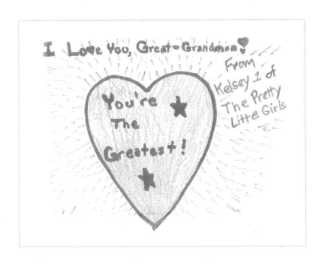

*"Kelsey's picture for Great-Grandmom"*

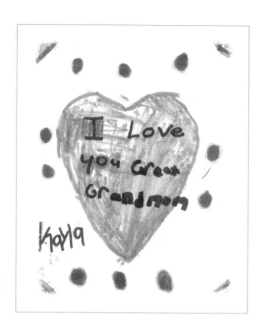

*"Kayla's picture for Great-Grandmom"*

Saying our meek good-byes to the staff, we left. I could not look back. I had just one thought to get in the car and get away.

It had already been planned that the girls and I were going to meet Karen, our daughter-in-law and their mother, in the early afternoon for lunch. The girls had won pizza coupons for participating in the library-reading program that they wanted to use. Kelsey, Kayla and I went into the restaurant and ordered their pizzas. When Karen arrived, she saw the state that I was in, so it was quickly decided that the girls would just carry out their food.

Outside the restaurant, we all hugged. Our treasured girls, Karen, Kelsey and Kayla were so kind to me. Karen's compassionate eyes and soft words, "Are you okay?" wrapped around me just like her sincere hug.

I retreated to my car, and waited for them to pull away. The key turned in the ignition and the roar that came from deep inside of me silenced the noise of the car's engine. This vehicle became like a private cave where I could let go all that was pent up inside of me. The screams and moans were gut wrenching. They did not have any familiar sound to me. Could they be coming from me?

Somehow, I was driving home, and the wails and screams continued. It was not like we were placing Charlotte somewhere else to live but more like dropping her off the end of the Earth.

Making it into the security of our own home, I fell to the floor and screamed and screamed, chastising myself for doing such a thing to Charlotte. I do not remember much more about that episode, but I cannot forget the bitter taste and the nauseous, sickening feeling that filled me.

I had read a long time ago that when a new sadness enters your life and you cry about it, the first few minutes of tears are for the present sadness and the rest of the tears that follow are for past sadness. Ray and I, like everyone, have had sadness in our life. The tears I shed for Charlotte's situation could have been cumulative, as the theory suggests. Maybe my heartbreak was intertwined, also, with a deep-rooted fear that one day this could happen to me. Whatever it all meant, I could not stop the sobs of remorse.

Ray was to pick his mom up at the center after work as usual and then take her to her new home. I could not bear to see it. I could not be there when Charlotte was left there. Ray found the courage to take his mother to her new residence that afternoon. It was done. Charlotte was there.

When Ray came into the house, he found me in our family room. We walked toward one another and fell into each other's arms. Ray's own sobs joined my sobs. We clung to each other. How my heart ached for him. As bad as it was for him, he still was so concerned about me and how hard this was for me. Ray's love for me is what gives me strength and courage to try and tackle the things I do. But this time I could not continue to battle. I had lost this war. I wanted to give Ray's mom what Ray had given to my dad and sister. I could not. Charlotte's circumstances made it impossible to have the more ideal solution.

Later that evening Ray and Matthew took Charlotte's chair to her. They found her in an aggressive and abusive state. She would not take her medicine and refused to eat. It took a while for Matthew to get the ice-cream-coated pills coaxed into Charlotte. She settled down somewhat after the meds kicked in, and Ray and Matthew slipped out without her noticing. It would not have done any good to tell her that they were leaving.

When Ray and Matthew got home and told me what had just happened, I believed that all my sadness was justified. It was not all right!

Visions of Charlotte's new living quarters haunted me that night. I could not sleep. Once again I made the nighttime march to Charlotte's room—only this time just to the doorway. I felt frozen to the spot. There was no locked gate, no chair, and no Charlotte. Oh, my God, what had we done! I left the emptiness of her room and made it back into our bed. The intercom was still by my pillow, but no sound of Charlotte was forthcoming. The silence was deafening.

Where was the tranquility I had hoped to find?

I could not go and see Charlotte the next day. Tears and sobs were still non-stop. Ray and I went for a short time on Saturday. I do not remember much except for my staunch feeling that—it still was not all right!

# ♥ Chapter Sixteen...

## Living with our Decision

*"Moving Charlotte out of our home was
something I never expected to happen.
It was part of succumbing to the reality of
living with Alzheimer's."*

I now had to live with our decision to place Charlotte in assisted-living, a decision I never wanted to make possible. I believed that we would always be able to give Charlotte all of the care that she would require.

Was I not able to have a somewhat normal life including getaways and vacations? Was I not managing and coping? Not being able to see the forest for the trees, I saw the life being sucked out of Charlotte but did not see the life being sucked out of me and us as I tried to do more than that of which I was capable. It was so difficult to take that unwanted step— to make that admission. It is indeed true; I am not Nancy Reagan. I had a lot of wonderful support at home with Ray and Matthew always offering a helping hand but no household staff. We are just an ordinary family who tried so hard to do the extraordinary, but Alzheimer's was just too much for us to manage anymore on our own. My hope for Charlotte living with us until the end died. Now my hope was for her to have the best quality of life that she could have in this tangled web of Alzheimer's.

The following Monday morning, I had to drop off some things for Charlotte at her new place. With much trepidation, I knocked on that door again. A smiling and apologetic woman in purple pajamas opened the door. It was the same woman who had let Kelsey, Kayla and me in a few days before when we had taken Charlotte's belongings to the facility. This woman was open and friendly, going on about things being hectic this morning and not having a chance to get dressed yet. Boy, I remembered that same kind of scenario happening to me just recently. My apprehension was being ever so slightly soothed by this scene. My heart actually stopped pounding in my throat. Did I have a slight grin on my face?

As I sheepishly looked around, this sunroom was how I remembered it the first time I visited this home—bright and large. The people around me seemed warm and friendly. I was able to hug the good woman in the purple pjs and thank her for all she was doing for Charlotte. Oh, thank you, Lord for this first step—a baby step maybe but a step forward.

I remembered the "Patient's Rights" paper that we received from the assisted-living facility and felt good about what it promised:

*Each participant and resident has the right to:*

*Be treated with consideration, respect, and full recognition of human dignity and individuality.*

*Receive care and services that are adequate and appropriate.*

*Privacy.*

*Be free from mental and physical abuse.*

*Be free from physical and chemical restraints.*

*Practice the religion of the resident's choice or to abstain from religious practice.*

*Be free from discrimination, as provided by state and federal law.*

*Consent or refuse consent to medical treatment.*

*Retain and use the resident's own personal property.*

*Receive and send unopened correspondence.*

*Private access to a telephone.*

*Unrestricted communication*

*—including personal visits with any person of the resident's choice.*[6]

This kind of care is what all of us wanted for Charlotte and it is the kind of care Charlotte is getting at her new residence. Do I call the new place Charlotte's home? No, I cannot say it is her "home." I say it is where Charlotte lives. It is not our home where her family planned for her to live out her days, but right now it is the best thing for her, for me and for us.

Are we involved with Charlotte? Indeed, we are! We are responsible for getting Charlotte to all of her doctor appointments and for making sure that she has all of her personal necessities. We also make all of her health care decisions and are very involved in the way in which her care is administered. We are responsible for her everyday living decisions but with many more hands to help with her physical care. So, to say the least, we did not drop Charlotte off and have little to do with her or for her. This was a surprise to some of our friends. They were not aware of how involved we would still remain in Charlotte's day-to-day care.

Charlotte would still continue to go to the adult day care center every weekday and enjoy all of the activities it had to offer. It was easier for me to visit Charlotte at the Center after she moved. It was very familiar territory for me, and all of us knew everyone there very well.

Then there was the assisted-living house. I had fought so hard not to make it a reality. It would take some time for me to accept it. It would have been the same with any unfamiliar facility where we would have placed Charlotte. It was just a part of the process of grieving for my unmet expectations. Moving Charlotte out of our home was something I never expected to see happen. It was part of succumbing to the reality of living with Alzheimer's.

Friends have shared concerns about their loved ones and the fears they have that their changing behavior might indicate Alzheimer's. It seems to me that getting old and dealing with some dementia is very different from Alzheimer's disease.

I was told that not all people who have dementia have Alzheimer's, but all people who have Alzheimer's do have dementia. I also was told that only after death and having the brain autopsied could they tell for sure if that person had Alzheimer's.

Wanting some definite answers to my never-ending questions, I often go over Charlotte's life and wonder if years of being on hormones or the fact that she had gone through electric shock therapy sometime during her second marriage could have had any bearing on her getting Alzheimer's.

In my layman's opinion, Charlotte's signs were so much more than confusion, repeating things, or forgetfulness. Charlotte seemed to lose the "know-how" of doing ordinary everyday things. She became unaware of the purpose for bathing. It did not occur to her to brush her teeth anymore. She had no sense of being stuffed or having a sick stomach, even after eating a five-pound box of chocolates. It was all so excessive.

To me Alzheimer's Disease inflicts so many bizarre behaviors on its victims that I have to keep reminding myself that part of the patient's brain is deteriorated. How would any one of us act if our intellect were not so finely tuned?

Living with someone with Alzheimer's forces you to look differently at your own life and at growing old. Forgetting names or facts or repeating myself sends a shiver down my spine. Is this the beginning for me? Having Ray not able to recall something can send an alarmed "Oh, no!" into my consciousness. When things like this happen, I must push the "what if" thought far from me. It could be paralyzing if I let it take hold.

When I think about our JR and Matthew having to take care of one of us if we get Alzheimer's, I have only one thought—please, Lord, allow the researchers to find the necessary medication to make life easier for the Alzheimer's patient and, of course, the cure. That is as far as I get. I just hope and pray that neither Ray nor I will suffer with this terrible disease and that our sons and daughter-in-law will not have to do for us what we have had to do for Charlotte.

*[Four million Americans have AD (Kawas 2003). Primarily as a result of the aging of the "baby boom" cohort, experts project the prevalence of AD to quadruple by 2050, "which means that 1 in every 45 Americans will be afflicted with the disease" (Kawas and Brookmeyer 2001). Nearly 85,000 Marylanders had AD in 2000 (Alzheimer's Association 2003). This number is expected to increase to nearly 195,000 by 2030 (Alzheimer's Association 2003).]*[1-6]

What will they do with all of us? Who will be able to care for us? How will they do it? My personal experience with Alzheimer's makes terminal cancer look like a much easier way to go.

The supplication for good health that I had begun to pray when I took care of Daddy changed. Since Charlotte was diagnosed with Alzheimer's, my prayer has been, "Lord, please bless Ray and me with healthy minds as we grow old." My fear is definitely saved for getting Alzheimer's. "Lord, please bless me as I grow older with a sound mind, even if my body has to fall apart." (Just a little bit of bargaining with God!)

Charlotte has been in her new place for almost three months, and it is hard for me to believe how fast that time has gone.

Visiting Charlotte now, I see how the assisted-living setting is truly better for her. There are many folks around to supervise her and pay attention to her all of the time. It is an upbeat place in spite of the circumstances that brought people there.

We do try to see Charlotte at least once a week there and look forward to maintaining a close and family-like relationship with the caring staff. We are indebted to them for giving Charlotte what we cannot. They take good care of Charlotte, and that is what really matters the most to us. Their goal is to give Charlotte the best quality of life that she can have in spite of having this unbearable disease. Our family shares that same goal for Charlotte.

Even in her self-imposed, isolated mindset, she has some signs of friendship among the group. One lady's face lights up when she sees Charlotte. I have seen this woman take Charlotte's hand and kiss it, to which Charlotte beams from the recognition. This gives me so much comfort and touches me deeply.

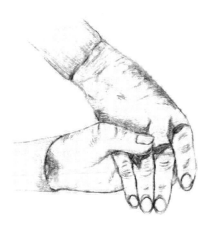

*"A new friend takes Charlotte's ringed hand"*

161

I continue to stop in at the adult day care center during the day to see how Charlotte is making out there. I still feel very close to the center's staff and appreciate all that they continue to do for Charlotte. They are a great team and there should be many, many more facilities like this to keep up with the growing population needing their kind of human services.

A result of the dedication of the caregivers at her new residence and their working so closely with the Alzheimer's center's staff is that Charlotte is sleeping at night. She is medicated in the evening with the anti-psychotic drug and a sleeping medication, Trazadone;[7] it works, and Charlotte is getting a full night's sleep. Together with the Alzheimer's facility, they also found that mixing Lorazapam[2] with Seroquel[4] does not work well. The smallest amount of Lorazapam[2] is only given as a last resort if she becomes agitated and aggressive. Now she is on the Seroquel[4] three times a day, which seems to be all that she needs to keep her calm.

The daytime meds are continually being fine-tuned and she does have bad days. One day when I visited Charlotte, she was having an off day and kept asking me to take her home. It was very difficult when she pleaded as she told me how mean "they" were to her. Even though I know that is not true, it still cuts deep into my being. I found myself reverting back to my old actions of looking for a distraction as I rounded up her animal book and video. I hoped that they would work. I wanted to save the day. I wanted to distract her from saying those things. I do not want Charlotte to say unkind or hurtful things, and I do not want others to be hurt by her words. I know that her new caregivers have feelings even though they are the professionals who definitely understand Alzheimer's, but all the same, I do not want Charlotte's negative behavior to be a barrier to getting good care.

I put the video in the player and brought her over to her chair, but it did not work this time. She had another UTI and was out of control again, causing havoc for her new caregivers. Distractions don't always work, and as our visit continued, she followed me with her eyes as I walked around the room. She was insistent that I take her home with me. I wanted to bundle her up and gather her things and do just that—bring her back home. I wanted to take her home so much, but I knew that I could not give her the care she needed.

We were advised not to bring Charlotte home for a visit. The staff said that Charlotte coming back to our house could confuse her and cause more distress for her. She may remember enough to know it as her home and refuse to leave. We could not take the risk that this might happen. It breaks my heart to think of her not spending her birthday or Christmas with us. I could not think about that then. It was just too sad.

The tears came once again as I quietly sneaked out the door and left by a different pathway so Charlotte could not see me leave. My grief resurrected, and I could not handle it. I could not call and check on Charlotte for several days. I am sure that there will be many times like this in the future, but it comes with the territory, as they say.

After all has been said and done, a few things have become clearer to me.

1. I now see how much sooner we needed to seek out the newer specialists— the geriatric physicians. We missed that opportunity early on because I did not understand the big picture at the time. It is only in hindsight that I can make this assessment. If we had done this, Charlotte may have had a grace period with new medications that would have made her staying with us manageable for a longer time.

2. Recently, while talking about this book with the geriatric specialist, who

first assessed Charlotte, I was questioned as to why I did not seek her out when things were so difficult for us. It took me a little while to ponder that question. I told her that in those in-between years when Charlotte was doing okay, I had forgotten about her specialty. In a most kind and gentle way, she assured me that it was a typical "caregiver syndrome" symptom—I was so focused on putting one foot in front of the other and being overwhelmed by all that was going on. Yes, it was a good question. Yes, it was a valid answer. Yes, it was an astute explanation.

3. Why did I not investigate or take advantage of the Alzheimer's hot line? I do not know!

Another aspect that I want to acknowledge is the neglect factor. No, I do not mean neglect of Charlotte—that never happened. I neglected some of my own needs over these last four years. A glowing example is a notice recently received from the radiologist reminding me that I have not had a mammogram since 2001. I have always been faithful to my yearly health checkups. Time just got away from me. I was consumed with Charlotte's needs and surely now have a tangible glimpse of how much I neglected myself and the rest of my family. This happens to many caregivers. More and more statistics show how vulnerable caregiver's health issues are because of the demands placed on them by the needs of the Alzheimer's patient.

I am reminded of the words, "Unless, you are fed, you cannot feed." It could also be said that, "Unless you are healthy, you cannot offer care to others."

## ♥ Chapter Seventeen...

### Making New Memories
*"Charlotte's ring now will be a part of my cherished wedding ring set, and I am so blessed to have this treasured memento."*

*Years:*
*Now and for as long as we have Charlotte*


A few days after Charlotte moved from our home, I was going through some of her things and came across some of her jewelry. I found the wedding band that Ray's dad had given to her. Looking down at this ring, I could not help but reminisce about another ring of long ago.

After my mother died, Daddy called us all together and said he was going to have a drawing for Mom's jewelry. Mom always was so fair-minded and at different times, she had joked about a drawing. There were four daughters and mom had four rings. Daddy gave each one of us a piece of paper with a number on it—a one, two, three or four. He then put mom's rings into his wide-brimmed hat and pulled them out one at a time. I had the number four on my slip of paper and the fourth ring pulled out was mom's wedding band. It was white gold, like my rings. Thrilled with my luck of the draw, I had Mom's ring welded to my engagement ring and wedding band. I have worn these rings like this for thirty years. I love having this tangible memento with me all the time.

Rather mindlessly, I slipped off the rings on my left hand and placed Charlotte's yellow gold wedding ring on my finger and then put my rings back on my finger. Charlotte's yellow gold ring did not match the others, but somehow it fit just fine. Ray's dad had given Charlotte this ring for their 25th wedding anniversary so that made it very special to me.

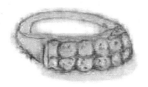

*"Charlotte's gold wedding band"*

I have a new insight. As I look at all of these rings together now, my mother's ring was a perfect match to my rings, just as we were a perfect match as mother and daughter. Charlotte's yellow gold ring is much more eye catching, just like Charlotte, and different from me. However in the greater scheme of things, they do fit together just fine. As soon as I can, I will have this ring welded to the others and the connection will be solid and complete. Charlotte's ring will be a part of my cherished wedding ring set, and I am so blessed to have this treasured memento. I will eat my words about Charlotte being a bit flashier than I am, as this cluster of rings is a little more glitz than I would chose; nonetheless, I will wear them with much affection. Their rings will always stir the remembrance of the endearing women who wore them before me.

The gate was taken down and put in the basement. Charlotte does not have the barrier of that gate anymore. I am so glad. That gate was the first concrete sign of her bondage into the disease that we know as Alzheimer's. That thought forces me to close my eyes and plead the silent prayer for the day that Charlotte is set free from her imprisonment.

However, it still surprises me, as I am working around the house and stop to look in Charlotte's empty room, that happy thoughts and flashbacks of the last months that Charlotte was home with us fill my mind. The memories are good ones that bring a smile to my face.

I remember things such as—

...Kelsey and Kayla looking through Charlotte's photo album with her—a little girl curled up on each side of her chair. She could not remember their name anymore, so Charlotte called them the "pretty little girls."

...The vision of our son, JR, playing bingo with his grandmother at the Center warms my heart as he does.

...Matthew's calling us to Charlotte's room to see one of Grandmom's getups with belts or scarves tied around her head with artificial flowers tucked in. I can almost hear Charlotte and Matthew laughing so hard with one another.

...I hear Charlotte's laughter as she watched "The Funniest Animals Show" on television. How she enjoyed that program.

...I think about Charlotte praising Ray for being so good to her. Yes, that did happen before and after the negative phase that she went through.

...I see Charlotte so excited to see and be with Marley-girl, as she called our dog.

...I actually laugh out loud as I remember the day Charlotte put on every red thing that she owned—two or three pairs of red socks, two pairs of red slacks, three red blouses, a red sweater, a red coat, a red hat and a pair of red gloves, to boot! How Charlotte and I laughed as I helped her to remove this all-red ensemble.

...I can even hear her thanking me for being so good to her. I was good to her. We have all been good to Charlotte and still are.

—These are the kind of memories I shall always treasure. These are the things our family will remember and tell over and over when we are together.

However,

It still is not all right!

It will never be all right!

Alzheimer's will never be all right!

Alzheimer's is stealing our loved one.

# *Epilogue*
## *March 2005*

Our journey with Charlotte continues...

Charlotte is in the latter stages of Alzheimer's disease. She still recognizes me but now thinks that I am her mother yet calls me Patti. Ray is no longer called by his name and only sometimes Charlotte says that he is her son. The words "pretty little girls" are a missing part of Great-Grandmom's vocabulary for Kelsey and Kayla; only her smile remains for them.

Charlotte's time at the adult day care center may be coming to an end. She is starting to display aggression and agitation while there; going there may be too much for her to handle anymore. This is so sad for Charlotte as she loved "going out," and now she will spend all of her time at the assisted living facility.

We do not know what tomorrow will bring. We only know that we still have to keep on making the best decisions that we can for Charlotte and be there for her as we, together, continue on this journey.

If you would like to share your story of caring for someone with Alzheimer's or helpful information that you have learned along the way, please visit my website lovespuntreasures.com or e-mail me at patti@lovespuntreasures.com

# Some Helpful Hints

Here is a copy of my "Helpful Hints" information that I prepared at the request of the nurses at the adult day care center:

Hopefully, by sharing strategies with one another, we can all learn to be more effective in handling the behavioral changes that occur in the person with dementia and/or Alzheimer's disease. In no way do these suggestions imply that we do things the "right way." The hints are about the way we try to handle everyday situations.

Some very practical actions we took and continue to take to help Charlotte as she enters into her own separate world are listed here. As her daughter-in-law and her caregiver, I found taking care of her on a daily basis reminded me of my days spent as a Kindergarten teacher. Being proactive gets better results than just being reactive. It can be very difficult dealing with her decreased capabilities. However, I find that when we recognize her mood changes right away, we are more likely to get her "smoothed over" and cooperative instead of anxious or aggressive.

Entertainment:
  ➢ Many television shows, including commercials, can create confusion for the person with dementia.

➢ Sports shows or better yet, tapes with animals and/or small children can be a source of enjoyment.

➢ "Baby Einstein" videos might be a good selection.

➢ Music, especially from their era can be soothing.

➢ Books with animal or baby pictures are a good choice.

➢ Children's coloring books offer another activity.

## Agitation:

At the first signs of agitation, WE react, before it escalates.

➢ Keep calm and redirect the person. Move the patient to another part of the room; offer a drink or snack.

➢ Rub the patient's arm and look him or her in the eye.

➢ Let the person feel your caring touch.

➢ Weather permitting, take the patient outside.

➢ When the patient is upset, accept those feelings. Do not deny the patient the right to express him or herself or try to talk the person out of his or her feelings. Listen with compassion.

➢ Giving the sufferer a large oval shaped lollipop to suck on has given over an hour of enjoyment instead of agitation in some of our situations.

## Wanting to take their clothes off:

> ➤ We found two useful items to help with this situation:
>
>> —A one-piece cover-up jumpsuit (beachwear) with zippered front, put on with the zipper in the back
>>
>> —Disposable painter cover-up with zippered front—put on with the zipper in the back—be sure to cut down the neckline to accommodate for reversing.

## Music at bedtime:

> ➤ MP3—CD player or one that can hold five or six CD's will play the entire night. In our case the player was on a remote control devise, so we could turn it off or on, when needed, from our bedroom.
>
> ➤ A baby intercom is a necessary item.

## Bedtime:

> ➤ Soft flannel sheets have a cozy feel to them.
>
> ➤ Very little light in the room eliminates shadows that can create fears, agitation or stimulation.

➢ Music playing might be soothing. (Observe their reaction and make sure that it is loud enough to grab the listener's attention.)

➢ It may be necessary to settle the patient down a few times before he or she is relaxed enough to fall off to sleep (turning the person to his or her preferred sleeping position, i.e., on the side, etc.,—rubbing back or arm)

➢ Staying with the person at first and assisting him or her with these types of things can help with a more restful sleep.

➢ Do very little talking.

➢ Position the person and say, "It is bedtime...close your eyes."

### Incontinence at Bedtime:

➢ It is important to prevent the person from lying in a wet bed. A cold, wet bed is a sure way to interrupt sleep as well as create skin irritations. It may take several attempts to find the right combination of diapering to be successful. It is worth the time and effort.

We have had success with the following:

➢ Pull-up with inner pad, vinyl pants covered with a diaper

➢ An extra large waterproof pad made from outdoor vinyl sold at fabric stores with a quilted cloth pad or disposable pad placed on top provide comfort and protection.

## Medications:

- ➤ Give only one NEW medicine at a time. Wait to see how the person reacts.
- ➤ Difficulty swallowing pills? Try putting in applesauce.
- ➤ Have a master list of daily medications.
- ➤ Dispense the meds listed and double check.
- ➤ Give meds from small medicine cups to ensure all pills are taken. Watch the person swallow them.

## Dehydration:

- ➤ Dehydration can increase agitation.
- ➤ Make sure the person drinks plenty of water.
- ➤ Avoid drinks with caffeine and water down juices to cut down on sugar intake.

## Infection:

- ➤ Watch for sudden behavioral changes, such as increased agitation or restlessness—these can be signs of infection, particularly of the urinary tract

➢ Notify the doctor immediately and give symptoms.

## Hospitalization:

➢ A word of caution for when the Alzheimer's patient is hospitalized: Many times, the hospital doctor will deem it necessary to lower or stop completely some of the drugs that have been giving relief from the patient's aggression and agitation. I have seen this send the patient into psychotic behavior and all of the misery that comes with that.

➢ Ask that the patient's regular physician be consulted before making any medicine adjustments or changes.

## Hygiene:

If the person toilets on his or her own:

➢ Remember to wash the patient's hands with soap and water as he or she most likely will not do a thorough washing. Pay attention to how well the patient can wipe himself or herself.

➢ Keep a supply of baby wipes and rubber gloves in the bathroom.

➢ DO NOT flush wipes down the toilet.

➤ Keep fingernails trimmed
   —Both patient and caregiver
➤ Keep bathroom free of harmful items

## Clothing:

➤ Pull on slacks with elastic waist
➤ Button front shirts
   —Person may be able to button
➤ Allow participation in dressing, as much as possible.
➤ Cotton socks to cushion feet
   —Many folks walk and pace frequently
➤ Snug fitting shoes w/non-skid soles.
➤ Remove or cut draw strings that hang from jackets or pants. They can get caught in objects and cause falls, etc.
➤ Keep minimal clothing, etc. where the patient has access


## Stairs:

➤ Going up
   —Stay behind the person and keep a firm hand on their back for support. Also, you can help lift up the patient by holding the waistband of the slacks.
➤ Going down
   —Use the "bottom bump" method (sitting on each step) or go in front and have the person put one hand on the railing and one hand on your shoulder to descend the steps. Make sure your

hands have a **FIRM** grip on handrail in case the patient gets a bit unsteady.

Keep a record:

> ➢ Keep a log of your loved one's day (in a notebook). Take it when going to the doctors so that you will not be saying "I am not sure when this or that took place." You will have confidence and feel competent in what you are doing for your loved one.

Children:

> ➢ Provide opportunities for the children in your family to interact with the Alzheimer's patient. Being in the presence of children seems to ignite a spark of reconnection to past times and, most of the time, brings many smiles and much joy to the patient.

> ➢ The children will benefit as much as the patient as this provides a great opportunity for children to experience first hand the many cycles of life. It teaches compassion and empathy for those who are elderly and failing.

If the children are not familiar with the patient, remember to prepare the children for the visit. Help them to understand what they might encounter with their family member. For example, their grandmother or grandfather may or may not recognize them, or might call them by someone else's name. They may not speak in clear sentences and the child may not be able to understand what they are saying—that is okay—the child only needs to smile. Their loved one may cry and seem sad—this, too, is part of life. Having the children involved with the Alzheimer's patient benefits everyone.

## Another good thing:

➢ Our family dog, Marley, gave Charlotte so much joy. She just loved to pet her and talk to her. Pets are a comfort to most of the elderly, even to a person who was fearful of animals earlier in their life.

## Be good to yourself:

➢ You don't have to give up everything you like to do—explore other ways to do them.

➢ If riding in a car is pleasurable for the person and you like taking rides on a Sunday afternoon, take rides and enjoy the change of scenery.

➢ If you like to walk for your exercise, get a wheelchair (on loan from the Lions Club) and push the patient on your walk (even if they are still ambulatory). You get a better workout, burn more calories and also can give the person a different setting. Good for both of you.

## Adult Day Care Centers:

I cannot say enough about adult day care centers. They are a great source of support for the caregiver. Knowing the staff and being able to have your loved one in their care is a relief for you and often for the patient too.

- ➤ Investigate resources to find the good ones; you need not ask the person if she wants to attend. Just take him or her.

- ➤ Be open and ask questions—share your ideas and concerns with the staff. They deal with patients with Alzheimer's and dementia everyday.

## The Department on Aging:

- ➤ Visit or call The Department on Aging in your county. They are another great resource. We have found a most caring group of individuals who work very hard on the behalf of the elderly. They have many suggestions for where to get help and how to get it.

## Respite Care:

- ➤ There are facilities that offer overnight respite care for your loved one.

➤ Investigate thoroughly and give them a try so that you can enjoy some rejuvenation time for yourself.

## Programs in your county:
➤ I can never say enough about the Department on Aging in Howard County, Maryland. The programs for the seniors are unbelievable. I would never have imagined how many options there were.

## Financial:
One aspect of this Alzheimer's journey that our family is living that I have not addressed is finances. I did not address this part because I do not have any real experience or much information to share with you. The area of finances is so involved and specific to each individual's circumstances that I had no basis on which to comment.

Charlotte is so fortunate to have a good health insurance plan. Also, she is in a financial position that makes it possible for her to receive assistance. When she attended the senior center plus facility and some of her time at the adult day care center, the fee was paid on a sliding scale per her income.

I know some families that have long-term health care insurance, and I just heard a blurb on the radio that veterans and their spouses may be entitled to some benefits for long-term care. However, my knowledge is limited. Each case is different. The only thing that I do know for sure is that Ray and I need to look into our own long-term "life plan" to know just where we stand. I do not look forward to this part of our journey even though I know how important it is. We also need to be more aware of legislation in our own state.

*State law can have a dramatic effect, for example, on whether a patient with AD can get needed services in the community instead of in a nursing home, a person with mild AD can continue to drive, or someone whose genes put the person at a higher risk of future AD can buy long-term care insurance. The right outcome on these and other public policy matters can make a real difference in the lives of AD patients and their families.* [1-7]

[1]- Curran, Jr., Schwartz, Policy Study On Alzheimer's Disease Care - Office of the Maryland Attorney General-Health Policy Development, January 2004

   [1-1]-Chapter 1 -Para. 2, Pgs. 1-2

   [1 2]-Chapter 1, Para.1, Pg. 1

   [1-3]-Chapter 1, Para. 1, Pg. 2

   [1-4]-Chapter 1, Para. 1, Pg. 2

   [1-5]-Chapter 1, Para. 2, Pg. 2

   [1-6]-Chapter 1, Para. 1, Pg. 5

   [1-7]-Preface, Para. 2, Lines 7-12, Pg. 1

[2]-Lorazapam - generic

[3]-Namenda-Forest Laboratories

[4]-Seroquel-AstraZeneca Phar.,LP

[5]-Steele, Kpounek, The Johns Hopkins University School of Medicine— Neuropsychiatry and Memory Group— Dementia Guideline Series for Families, 2nd Ed. 1999

   [6]-Group Senior Assisted Housing Resident's Rights—MD Office on Aging

   [7]-Trazadone - generic

# Resources

## Alzheimer's Association
www.alz.org          (800) 272-3900
- ➢ Provides information to find local chapters
- ➢ Contact Center is available 24 hours
- ➢ Seven days a week

## Alzheimer's Disease, Education & Referral Center  (ADEAR)
www.alzheimers.org   (800) 438-4380
- ➢ A service of the National Institute on Aging

## Eldercare Locator
www.eldercare.gov   (800) 677-1116
- ➢ Eldercare Locator Assistance for locating local, state and community resources.
- ➢ Hours:  M - F,  9:00 a.m. – 8:00 p.m.

## National Institute on Aging (NIA)
www.nia.nih.gov    (800) 438-4380
- ➢ NIA is the primary federal agency on Alzheimer's disease research at the National Institutes of Health